An Essential Guide to Caring for People with a Learning Disability and Autistic People

This essential text presents the core information that all nursing students and apprentices along with other key health and social care professions, regardless of field, need to know about caring for people with a learning disability and autism. It outlines some of the key challenges faced by people with a learning disability and autism, and ways in which good care can improve their quality of life. People with a learning disability and autism are more likely to need support with aspects of everyday life, be marginalised within society, including within health and social care, and die younger than the rest of the population. They are also more likely to have additional communication needs, sensory processing difficulties and require significant support to access healthcare as well as other opportunities across the course of their lives.

This innovative text highlights the core knowledge that all health and social care professionals need and emphasises the benefits of learning across different fields of practice. It presents information about common conditions, key skills, and where a standard approach may need to be changed when caring for a person with a learning disability and autistic people. It demystifies key issues and commonly misunderstood concepts and topics including distressed behaviours, consent and reasonable adjustments. The book also focuses on addressing health inequalities, improving communication, understanding mental capacity and presents case studies throughout to illustrate how care can and should be delivered.

Written for all who aspire to understand the needs of these individuals and to deliver care as effectively as possible, this collaborative text brings together the voices of services users and their families and carers, with those of nurses, other health professionals, lecturers, and nursing students and apprentices.

Helen Jones is a registered nurse for people with a learning disability and currently Head of Learning Disability and Autism at Birmingham and Solihull Mental Health Foundation Trust.

Andrea Page is a registered nurse for people with a learning disability and Associate Professor at Birmingham City University.

Samantha Salmon is a registered nurse for people with a learning disability and Senior Lecturer at Birmingham City University.

An Essential Guide to Caring for People with a Learning Disability and Autistic People

Enabling a Cross-Field Approach

Edited by Helen Jones,
Andrea Page and Samantha Salmon

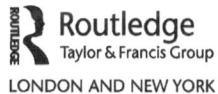
Routledge
Taylor & Francis Group

LONDON AND NEW YORK

Cover image: Designed by a user of the learning disability services in Birmingham

First published 2025
by Routledge
4 Park Square, Milton Park, Abingdon, Oxon OX14 4RN

and by Routledge
605 Third Avenue, New York, NY 10158

Routledge is an imprint of the Taylor & Francis Group, an informa business

British Library Cataloguing-in-Publication Data
A catalogue record for this book is available from the British Library

ISBN: 978-1-032-37759-9 (hbk)
ISBN: 978-1-032-37758-2 (pbk)
ISBN: 978-1-003-34176-5 (ebk)

DOI: 10.4324/9781003341765

Typeset in Bembo and Helvetica Neue LT Pro
by KnowledgeWorks Global Ltd.

Access the Support Material: www.routledge.com/9781032377582

The editors would like to dedicate this book to every person with a learning disability and autism. We believe that everyone deserves equitable and effective care as well as respect and the right to have their voices heard. We would also like to extend this dedication to student nurses and apprentices from the fields of learning disability, adult, children's and mental health nursing across the United Kingdom.

Contents

Section 2: Lived experiences and professional insights: Understanding care and treatment for people with learning disabilities and autistic people   **33**

About the editors

Dr Helen Jones

Helen is Head of Learning Disability and Autism at Birmingham and Solihull Mental Health Foundation trust, a position she has held since February 2024. Prior to this she was a senior lecturer at Birmingham City University where she worked between 2011 and 2024.

Helen is a learning disability nurse and has always had a special interest in areas including forensic nursing, epilepsy, and legal and ethical frameworks within learning disability nursing. Helen's research for both her MSc and her PhD focused on the experiences of women with learning disabilities within secure care and forensic services. As part of her PhD studies Helen began to embrace and develop her knowledge around feminist research approaches which she used to frame her methodological approaches. This was to help ensure she could more carefully capture the voices of people with a learning disability, something she feels very passionate about and continues to champion within her current role in the NHS.

Dr Andrea Page (orcid.org/0000-0001-5699-4786)

Andrea is Associate Professor at Birmingham City University, a position she has held since August 2015. Prior to this she was a senior lecturer and has worked at the university since November 2000.

Throughout her career she has always had an interest in how challenging behaviours are managed. As a direct result of her masters, parents and siblings of children and adults with a learning disability who present with challenging behaviours are now taught breakaway techniques. She continues to advocate for this through her partnership working and teaching. Andrea's PhD research looked at holding children for clinical procedures. This led to a website on clinical holding techniques being developed, which you can access and share. Her interest in preventing postural distortion began as a student nurse and has continued to develop as professional knowledge in this area has continued to expand.

Samantha Salmon (orcid.org/0009-0001-0039-3225)
Samantha is Senior Lecturer in Learning Disability Nursing at Birmingham City University and Senior Fellow of Advance HE. She is Admissions Tutor for Learning Disability Nursing and Deputy Course Lead for the Future Nurse Curriculum. Through her roles, Samantha has empowered staff, students and apprentices from all fields of nursing to better meet the needs of people with a learning disability and championed the voice of learning disability nursing students and apprentices. She has a special interest in postural care; it was through a meeting with Andrea Page and Sarah Clayton many years ago as a student that Samantha first heard about the statistics within the CIPOLD (2013) report and avoidable deaths of people with a learning disability, and this was the catalyst to wanting to raise awareness in other fields. She recognises the importance of supporting students and valuing their previous skills and experiences to encourage them to develop to meet their potential and identify how they can make positive changes in practice.

Notes on contributors

Dr Stefan Cash, Senior Lecturer at Birmingham City University. In 2012, Stefan was awarded The Queen's Nurse Award as recognition for his outstanding dedication to the health service. Stefan's specialities include clinical simulation, paediatric accident and emergency, paediatrics, child health and children's nursing.

Kate Chadwick, BSc (Hons) Therapeutic Radiography, MSc oncology practice. Senior lecturer in radiography – health professions. Kate is part of the Bronchiolitis guideline development group and has ongoing involvement in NIHR-funded study (UK wide open-label randomised clinical trial of respiratory support in infants with acute bronchiolitis). She is a member of the West Midlands Review Oversight Panel (ROP) to review completed LeDeR reviews and a member of the DSMIG where evidence-based practice healthcare for people with Down syndrome is developed. She is a "Treat me well" champion with Mencap. Her doctoral studies started in 2022 and she is looking at 'A grounded theory and narrative inquiry investigation into the equity of access to radiotherapy treatment for people with learning disability and/or autism'.

Dr Helen Clarke, Admission tutor for Biomedical Science, Birmingham City University. Her degree is in Applied and Human Biology and her PhD focuses on the effects of Metformin on the vascular system. She joined BCU in 2003 and embarked on her teaching career in health education. She teaches on clinical courses to midwives, child and neonatal nurses, and is also involved with the Biomedical Sciences degree with admissions, teaching modules and as deputy course lead

Sarah Clayton, CEO Simple Stuff Works Associates. Sarah has managed her own successful business for over 20 years developing and delivering nationally recognised accredited training in protection of body shape and measurement of body symmetry. As a company Simple Stuff Works (SSW) provides effective, night-time positioning solutions for people with complex healthcare needs. SSW provides accredited training and support for Allied Health Professionals (AHPs) across both community and acute teams. SSW are world renowned for their knowledge and expertise in the field of therapeutic positioning.

Sarah Davies, Lecturer: FdSc Nursing Associate Degree programme, Birmingham City University. Sarah has worked as a nurse in community and inpatient settings for adults with learning disabilities and within more general inpatient settings before joining Birmingham City University in July 2022. As a nursing student, Sarah presented at national conferences and worked as a mentor and student ambassador for the university representing learning disability nursing. She achieved the Health and Social Care Award for Student Practice at the end of her studies. Since joining the university Sarah has undertaken a variety of professional qualifications and is looking forward to starting her Master's in Public Health as well as continuing her work as an External Examiner.

Elisha Deegan, PhD candidate, Western Sydney University. Elisha first contacted Andrea Page in 2016, to explore Basic Life Support Training for people with a distorted body shape. Since then Elisha has gone on to gain a Masters at the University of Tasmania, Australia. Her research looked at disability-specific resuscitation and basic life support which has led to several further papers being published.

Sally-Anne Dicken, Community Learning Disability Nurse, South Worcestershire Community Learning Disability Team. At the time of writing Sally-Anne has been shortlisted across several categories for the Student Nursing Times Awards. She is the founder of the Makaton LDND group. Sally-Anne trained at Birmingham City University.

Farzana Follows, a Registered Nurse (RNLD), Farzana is a Clinical Commissioning Manager – Learning Disabilities and Autism, Coventry and Warwickshire Partnership NHS Trust. Farzana has experience of working with people with a learning disability detained under the Mental Health Act in a mental health hospital, supporting them from admission through to discharge, and working with services in the community to prevent unnecessary admissions to a mental health hospital for people with a learning disability and autistic people. Her current role involves supporting the aims of the Learning Disability and Autism programme in preventing unnecessary admissions and supporting timely discharges from mental health hospitals. She oversees local arrangements for the Dynamic Support Register, Care (Education) and Treatment Reviews and Local Area Emergency Protocol meetings as well as offering support to the keyworker service commissioned as part of the programme to work with children, young people and their families.

Amanda Glennon, CEO Inclusive Teaching (IT) Matters, Amanda is an ambassador at the Makaton Charity and has been a Makaton tutor for over ten years supporting individuals, families and organisations to remove communication barriers. Amanda has co-produced many resources and projects across healthcare, which have included winners of the Nursing Times Awards and the Patient Safety Awards. Amanda is a regular speaker at national conferences and previously spent her early career in senior roles for global organisations. She credits her family, in particular her daughter who has a learning disability, as her inspiration.

Anna Goldsmith, BA Hons., Director and Founder of Simple Stuff Works Associates, specialist in therapeutic positioning training and care. As a company, Simple Stuff Works (SSW) provides effective, inexpensive night time positioning solutions for people with complex healthcare needs. Alongside award winning equipment SSW provides accredited training and support for AHPs across both community and acute teams. Trading internationally SSW are world renowned for their knowledge and expertise in the field of therapeutic positioning.

Ruth Hirst, Lecturer in learning disability nursing, Birmingham City University. Ruth worked as a nurse in specialised community and inpatient settings for adults with a learning disability before joining Birmingham City University in March 2022. Her nursing roles include working in a forensic inpatient service caring for women with a learning disability and as a community nurse providing early intervention and intensive support to adults with learning disabilities in the community. As a nursing student, Ruth was part of a professional student nurse networking group that promoted the benefits of online networking. Ruth co-authored her experience of this in the journal *Learning Disability Practice*.

Sheryl King, Lecturer in learning disability nursing, Birmingham City University. Sheryl joined the University in October 2020. Her career has predominantly been spent supporting adults and children with learning disabilities in the community in a variety of locations around the West Midlands. Her roles have included Community Nursing within a multi-disciplinary team, Community Team Worker at Acorns Children's Hospice, Special School Nursing and Community LD Nurse in a Child & Adolescent Mental Health Team. Sheryl has studied over the years at BCU and in addition to her Registered Nurse qualification she has achieved her BSc in Community Health Nursing and a Graduate Certificate in Mental Health Studies. In conjunction with her lecturer role, she is also Deputy Admissions Tutor for the Learning Disability Nursing Course.

Dr Andrew McDonnell, Consultant Clinical Psychologist to and Director of Studio III Clinical Services; Director, clinical consultant and Team Leader to Studio III Training and visiting professor in Autism Studies at Birmingham City University. He has a special interest in arousal mechanisms in people with autism and the management of severe challenging behaviours. Other areas of interest are stress management, person-centred approaches to behaviour management, arousal mechanisms and their application to human behaviour, and sensory perceptual processing differences. Dr McDonnell has been involved with several undercover documentaries and is considered an expert in the complex reasons why abuse occurs and in supporting vulnerable people traumatised by their experiences within care systems.

Katie Meah, Assistant Professor and Course Director for Learning Disabilities Nursing – MSc at Coventry University. She has worked in a number of roles and settings as a learning disability nurse since qualifying and as a health visitor after gaining her SCPHN qualification. Katie undertook additional training to become a senior reviewer for LeDeR for NHS Birmingham and Solihull Clinical Commissioning Group and has been instrumental in sharing and informing learning with academics and students to better equip them to recognise their role in identifying and reporting premature deaths in people with a learning disability or autism.

Victoria Moloney, Lecturer in learning disability nursing, Birmingham City University. Victoria joined the university in 2022 having gained a wealth of experience in assessment and treatment, short-term breaks, community and specialist nursing. Victoria was a continuing healthcare assessor for people with learning disabilities which involved the assessment and collation of information for Decision Support Tool (DST) meetings and making recommendations regarding funding needs and if personal health budgets. Her most recent clinical role was as team manager and named nurse for children in care. The role also included training others including carers in the statutory requirements in meeting health needs and supporting identified needs or signposting to other appropriate professionals. The role of named nurse meant oversight of all the children in care and liaising with local, regional and national agencies depending on where the child or young person was placed.

Joe Powell, Chief Executive of All Wales People First. Joe was diagnosed with Asperger Syndrome in 1996. His experiences as a user of services and his journey from England to Wales where he is now Chief Executive of All Wales People First is documented in Section 2. All Wales People First is a National Umbrella body for self-advocacy groups for people with learning disabilities in Wales. They believe that self-advocacy is the most important form of advocacy and want to bring about real change for members so that they can be active and contributing citizens.

Melanie Wakeman, Mel was a lecturer in nutrition and applied physiology, curriculum lead and course director from 1997 until 2017 at Birmingham City University. She now runs her own business concentrating on distressed eating, eating disorder recovery, menopause nutrition and wellbeing.

Alison Warren, Academic Lead for Practice Learning, Practice Learning Experiences: Development and Creation. She has a wealth of experience in Children and Young People's (CYP) Nursing, and has worked in a number of roles including Education Fellow for Health Education England (HEE) Clinical Matron for Children's Services, PICU, Neurosciences, Hepatology and Liver Transplantation, Orthopaedic' s, CYP Clinical Education, Skills and Simulation, Preceptorship Lead and Resuscitation services. In 2014–15 Alison worked with a small project team for Health Education West Midlands on the 'Every Student Counts' project and is a co-author of the 'Mind the Gap – Exploring the needs of early career nurses and midwives in the workplace' report. Alison is a founder member and Chair of the West Midlands Regional Preceptorship Group and has participated in the development of the National Preceptorship Framework (2022) where she sits on the West Midlands Interim Quality Mark Panel. Alison is also the Chair of the Partners in Paediatrics (PiP) Senior Nurse Forum.

Anna Waugh, Director and Founder of Simple Stuff Works Associates, specialist in therapeutic positioning training and care. As a company Simple Stuff Works (SSW) provides effective, inexpensive night-time positioning solutions for people with complex healthcare needs. Alongside award winning equipment SSW provides accredited training and support for AHPs across both community and acute teams. Trading internationally SSW are world renowned for their knowledge and expertise in the field of therapeutic positioning.

Linda Woodcock, Director of AT-Autism and Head of Families and Support. Linda is also a parent of an adult with autism and severe and complex needs. Linda has many years' experience of working with individuals with autism and their families. She previously managed advice and advocacy services and a family support service for a large regional charity. She has been instrumental in devising and delivering innovative person–centred training courses for parents and families in understanding autism and behaviours that challenge.

Student nurses – BSc (Hons)/MSci in learning disability nursing pathway: Emmie Jeffrey (at time of contribution, Emmie was a first-year student nurse); Jamie White (at time of contribution, Jamie was a third-year student nurse); Taiwo Sanni (at time of contribution, Taiwo was a first-year student nurse); Blessing Taiwo (at time of contribution, Blessing was a second-year student nurse); Jemima Tandoh (at time of contribution, Jemima was a first-year student nurse).

Learners studying at Birmingham City University through the Registered Nurse Degree Apprenticeship pathway: Christine Cooper (at time of contribution Christine was in her second year of her studies). At the time of their contribution, all of the following apprentices were in their final year of study: 09/21 SO cohort (Sonia Allibone, Nikita Garrick, Debbie Marsh and Lee Vessey), 09/20 4 year cohort (Olumide Dada and Baldwin Ngambi), 09/22 SO cohort (Jose Ferin).

Foreword

The <u>NHS Constitution</u> has six values, which says by living these values, we can ensure the best possible care for patients:

1   Working together for patients

2   Respect and dignity

3   Commitment to quality of care

4   Compassion

5   Improving lives

6   Everyone counts

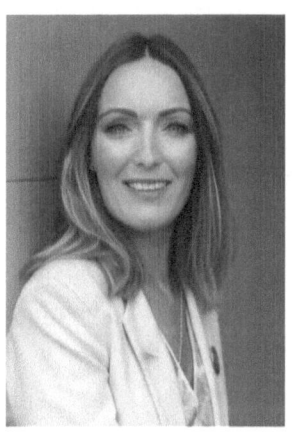

FIGURE 1 Paula McGowan, OBE

The overriding evidence from the learning disability mortality review and Mencap's various campaigns has told us that these important values do not always exist for autistic people and those who have a learning disability. LeDeR has highlighted persistent shocking inequalities, with women dying 26 years younger than those in the general population and men 22 years younger.

My teenage son Oliver is amongst these statistics. Oliver's avoidable death shone a light on exactly why his training is essential. The training is named after him. In brief, Oliver was a very popular youngster who was loved and admired by so many people. Oliver had a diagnosis of cerebral palsy, epilepsy, autism and a mild learning disability.

However, Oliver's disabilities did not hold him back, he had a steely determination to overcome any barriers that he faced. He played for the England FA football development teams, He was ranked third best in the country for 200 metres and was being trained for the Paralympics team. He passed his GCSEs and Btec examinations. Oliver was incredibly artistic and loved painting and drawing.

Despite his incredible achievements Oliver is dead. He died because clinicians didn't listen to him, his parents or other professionals who were working with him daily and knew him well.

Oliver was admitted to hospital having focal seizures. Horrifically he was given an antipsychotic to help treat his anxiety when in seizure. Oliver was not mentally unwell. It was written in the drug charts in the allergy box that Oliver was allergic to all forms of antipsychotic medication. Yet it was administered, it caused Oliver's brain to swell so badly, we were told it was coming out of the base of his skull. Oliver died an awful and avoidable death

I do not believe that any clinician goes into the caring profession wanting to cause harm or distress to their patients, I believe they want to be able to care and support their patients to the best of their ability.

Sadly, the truth is that huge numbers of staff simply do not have the knowledge or skills in caring and treating neurodiverse patients. They do not have knowledge in understanding exactly what neurodiversity is and how it affects the individual person. There is unconscious bias and at times prejudice, which leads to diagnostic overshadowing, which can have catastrophic outcomes for these communities. Staff do not have skills to make reasonable adjustments; many do not understand why these adjustments must be made. Neurodiverse people have told us that staff do not have the skills to communicate with them, they are not skilled in adapting their language to meet their individual needs and they do not understand perceived challenging behaviour as a person trying to communicate their needs.

I am therefore delighted to write a foreword for this wonderful book that has been written for our nurses in training to tackle some of the above issues that people who have a learning disability and autistic people face when coming into our hospitals. I am pleased that the book covers key challenges faced by people with learning disabilities and the way in which nurses across all fields of nursing can aim to improve their quality of life.

These are:

■ Better physical care for people with profound and multiple learning disabilities

■ Key legal challenges and how nurses can support and understand these

■ Conditions that are more prevalent or may present differently in people with learning disabilities, demonstrating current and evidence-based practices within these.

Having this knowledge will certainly give our nursing staff the necessary skills to ensure that they are able to support and care for neurodivergent patients, so that good healthcare outcomes will be achieved.

It is wonderful to see that real stories have been included in this book. It is essential that the voices of experts by experience are heard and learned from. This is the way to changing what has gone before, changing culture, hearts and minds.

Paula McGowan OBE

Foreword

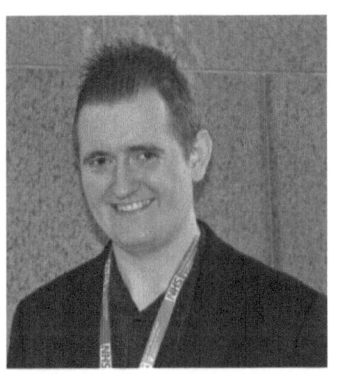

It is really welcome to see continued focus both in terms of research and new insights for the branch of learning disability nursing. This new textbook will further enhance the opportunities to understand how to deliver better care of those with a learning disability and autistic people alongside the expertise of learning disability nurses.

Central to this is co-production and design and engagement to support better services for those who need them. That is why I'm delighted to join you writing this foreword and wish to introduce Carl:

FIGURE 2 Carl Shaw, learning disability and autism advisor, NHS England

My name is Carl Shaw, I have a mild learning disability and am employed at NHS England as a Learning Disability and Autism Adviser. People with a learning disability and autistic people have worse health outcomes than the general population. For example, the average age of death for people with a learning disability is 65 and 49 per cent of those deaths are from avoidable causes. It is also common that people with a learning disability are prescribed psychotropic medication when they do not have a diagnosed mental health condition; this is often to manage what people deem as challenging behaviour. Considering all of this, it is important that people with a learning disability get access to their annual health check and that this is done to a high standard with a health action plan, that people get good-quality medication reviews where a person's whole life is thought about, and that services are aware and implement what reasonable adjustments people need. It's also important to know that people with a learning disability are human beings with individual needs and that all individuals are different. The best advice I can give you is to get to know the people you are caring for and you will see that we are like everyone else.

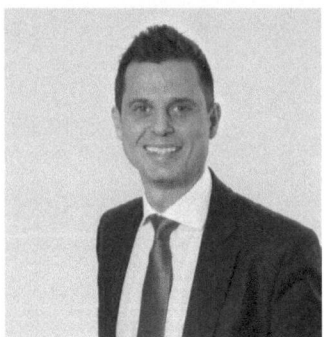

FIGURE 3 Professor Mark Radford,
CBE

'Carl really does highlight some of the known issues and challenges. The UK is unique in having this branch of nursing which has shown phenomenal change and further developments to support care and develop the profession' (Professor Mark Radford CBE, Chief Nurse of Health Education England and Deputy Chief Nursing Officer for England).

Foreword

Listening and learning with and from student healthcare practitioners is at the core of what we do as healthcare educators; each of us comes from our own speciality and share willingly the how and why to care for an individual who brings a different 'script' to your care arena.

As student nurses studying together it is important that you acknowledge the 'corporate identity of the registered nurse' and, by that, I mean the shared skill base you all have: you have all studied the same modules and now it's about exploring how you take those skills into your own field of destination. But! The lesson that needs to be learnt relates to applying your skill in your care arena to individuals who are often marginalised and maybe you have not had either consistent or positive exposure to during your career journey so far.

Learning disability nurses are great sharers; we consistently listen to the vibe of our tribe to both make a difference and ensure people with a learning disability get what you and I take for granted. We are the smallest field of nursing but have a proven track record of demonstrating that in healthcare if you can get it right for someone who has a learning disability you can get it right for everybody. It's about that philosophy of seeking non-traditional sustainable solutions to issues others think are insurmountable.

So, think about it! You would find out who the tissue viability nurse was in your hospital, or the perinatal mental health nurses, so why not the learning disability nurse? We all work in busy arenas but by working in a joined-up way then we demonstrate that 'together we are better' and that every patient matters.

Whether your qualification takes you into medicine, social care or nursing care you need to listen to each other and talk to each other. This book provides you with a springboard for those conversations in the spirit of appreciative enquiry and reinforces a catalyst for change – use it.

Twenty years ago I set out to facilitate a conference; Positive Choices fast became the life blood for student nurses studying towards a learning disability nursing qualification – especially as it gave them the chance to be in the majority rather than the minority in a professional group setting.

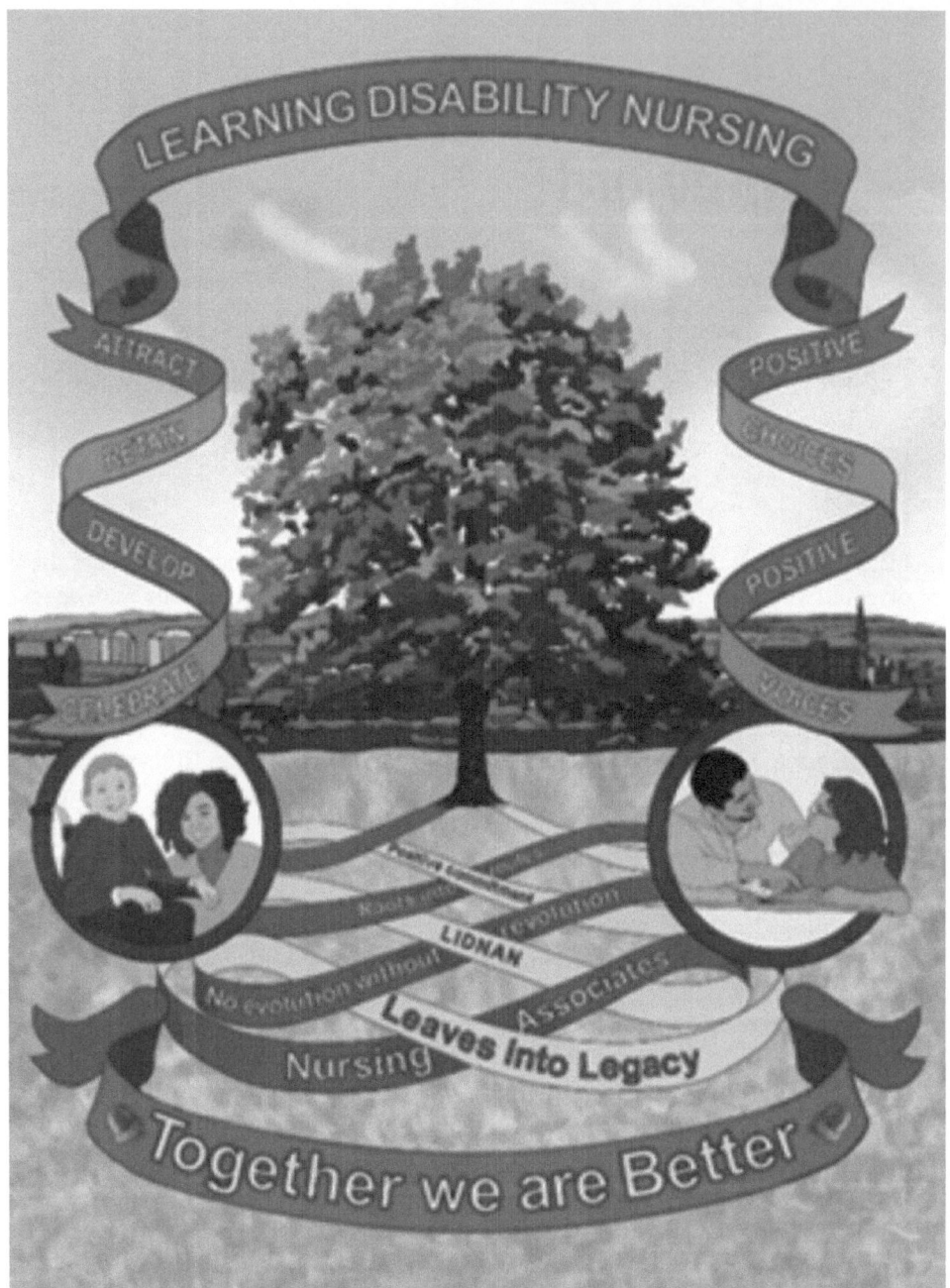

FIGURE 4 Positive Choices image designed by Tony Wade

This booked-out event happens every year thanks to the dedication of a small team of academics who fundraise, plot and persuade people to give of their time and talents to ensure the event remains free to all delegates. The first event was held in Nottingham in response to the negative experiences learning disability students were experiencing in the wider health community and is now the biggest student nurse conference across the UK and Ireland.

So why did I do it?

In 2004 a group of my students went to a national event: they were told:

Why did you bother with learning disability?

Is it too late for you to change branch?

You should have done mental health.

There's no future in it.

No one's really interested in learning disability nursing.

For some of us, learning disability nursing has always been a positive choice, one made as a conscious decision at the start of our careers; for others it's something that came along by chance following practice experience or a chance encounter. Whatever the path that took the individual into learning disability nursing it is a career path that requires great resilience.

We (nursing) are an evolving profession; we develop alongside science and society, but in learning disabilities it's often that bit quieter: changes in policy, philosophy and attitude often see the role of the Registered Nurse Learning Disabilities (RNLD) marginalised and its existence called into question, and when things go wrong in a small area (no matter how big that wrong is) the debate about the future and benefit of the RNLD is raised again.

Positive Choices is a thriving network/information exchange/social forum/support mechanism and conference that for the last 20 years has brought together student nurses, academics, movers and shakers in the learning disability world, people who have a learning disability and those who love them to a 500-place, free-to-access, two-day conference. We have made a difference! You can too.

Helen M. Laverty MBE
Professional lead for Learning Disability Nursing, Faculty of
Medicine and Health Sciences, University of Nottingham

Preface

This book aims to provide nurses in higher education, especially those who have chosen adult, child or mental health nursing and other health and social care professionals who are not learning disability trained with core knowledge.

- People with a learning disability are more likely to have communication needs that are different.

- People with a learning disability are more likely to have comorbidities and experience inequalities.

- Although you may already be knowledgeable and skilled there may be a need for you to change your approach when supporting a person with a learning disability.

With the introduction of the Future Nurse programme (and Nursing Associate) and the loss of a learning disability nursing route in some universities in England this is an ideal time to develop supporting literature for students who may not have access to specific teaching and practice opportunities relating to learning disability. This is a collaborative book written with a range of professionals, academics and learning disability student nurses/apprentices. The book will use case studies, threaded throughout the book to support discussions within chapters.

In summary, this book focuses on practical tips to help you to support a person with a learning disability within your field of practice. If you are supporting someone with a learning disability, this book will provide you with insight and tips on what you could do differently.

Acknowledgements

The editors of this book would like to express their heartfelt thanks to the following people, without whose skill and support this book would not have happened:

All contributors: Thank you for your knowledge and the time you have dedicated to writing this book around your existing commitments – we appreciate all of you.

Lisa Barker: We are forever grateful for your incredible artwork and for working with us to produce the front cover.

Matt Kelly: Thank you for your skill, support and patience in creating the illustrations within the book.

Dr Simon Cook (BCU ADD): Thank you for your support given to the nurse apprentices for their section and chapters.

And a huge thank you to our publishers for supporting us through this process – we have loved working with you.

Why have we written this book?

1

The people who inspired this book

Helen Jones, Samantha Salmon and Andrea Page

Below we have outlined chosen case studies that reflect the experiences of real people with a learning disability and their families. Unfortunately there are many more we could have chosen and that have also inspired this book. The care and treatment that Tony, Rachel, Thomas and Laura received reflect the need for *all* health and social care professionals to understand more about people who have a learning disability and autistic people. We must also remember the experiences of Oliver McGowan as told by his mother, Paula, in her foreword for this book. When using and reading this book to inform and support your own practice and learning please do remember these people and their lives.

Tony Hickmott

On 31 October 2022, Tony Hickmott left Cedar House, a mental health facility near Canterbury in the UK for the last time. He had been detained under Section 3 of the Mental Health Act (1983, amended 2007). Tony was eventually detained there for 21 years, four months and three days. Due to his profound learning disabilities and autism it was reported that it had become increasingly difficult for his parents to meet Tony's needs at home. His detention is reported to be even sadder as his increasing anxiety and aggression at home could not be supported through local community provision and led to his detention and use of the Mental Health Act. Cedar House was a four-hour round-trip from his family and yet, despite this, his parents made the trip every week for the entire time he was detained except during the COVID-19 pandemic. In 2009 Tony was made subject to long-term segregation as defined under the Mental Health Act. This meant he was confined to a small area consisting of a bedroom, toilet and living room. This also meant being isolated from any other people living within the hospital and lack of meaningful and therapeutic activity. Long-term segregation legally requires assessment, review and scrutiny. Despite this Tony remained in long-term segregation until he was discharged in October 2022. During this time it is also reported that

DOI: 10.4324/9781003341765-2

approaches such as the use of antipsychotic medication and restraint were used to manage Tony within this setting.

Although Tony was identified and assessed as being able to leave hospital in 2013, an appropriate package of care could not be found. There appear to have been several failings including the failure of the local authority and Integrated Care Board to find an appropriate package of aftercare for Tony, packages of care being proposed that were too restrictive and the decision not to offer Tony a Community Treatment Review, all of which are legal requirements under the Mental Health Act.

In 2019 media scrutiny began when Tony's parents failed to get the support and change that they needed for Tony to be able to leave hospital. In the short term this media scrutiny posed a risk that Tony would have to leave Cedar House and be moved even further away. In the meantime, with legal support Tony's parents along with further media support began to effect the change that was so needed for Tony. An application was made to the Court of Protection and despite some additional hurdles relating to identifying appropriate packages of care, the legal requirements set out by the Court of Protection meant that discharge planning was more rigorously monitored until Tony left the hospital. With the help of local housing providers, care providers and NHE England Tony was able to move into his own home near his family and with a package of care that better supported his needs. This included well-trained staff to care for Tony.

Tony's family and those that have fought for his right to live independently in the way that he wishes will inspire change and further support for community provision for people with learning disabilities and/or autism who are 'stuck' within mental health facilities without the care that they need.

Consider Tony when reading chapters that include the following:

- Autism and Learning Disabilities
- Mental Health Act Reform
- Over use of [antipsychotic] medication (STOMP)
- Community Treatment Reviews and the Mental Health Act (1983)
- Mental Capacity Act (2005) and Deprivation of Liberty Safeguards (2009)
- NHS Long Term Plan (2019) and the reduction of Long Term Segregation and Seclusion targets
- Low-arousal techniques and managing behaviours that challenge

Rachel Johnston

Rachel Johnston died in 2018 following the extraction of all of her teeth. This procedure was recommended following a dental inspection of her teeth earlier that year where it was identified that Rachel was at risk of infection. Rachel was 49 years old, living at Pirton Grange Care Home near Worcester. She was described as a happy person who loved life and her family. Rachel had physical and learning disabilities and needed support with many elements of daily care and living. This included brushing and caring for her teeth.

Rachel began to deteriorate physically following discharge from the hospital, four hours after the operation had taken place. Over the following 48 hours she bled intermittently from her mouth and never fully woke during this time. When the ambulance was called two days after the operation had occurred Rachel died shortly afterwards.

The LeDeR Mortality Review into Rachel's death questioned the risk of carrying out this operation on someone who has severe learning and physical disabilities. Mention was made of communication between professionals and the dental care received prior to the operation. In addition to this it appears that the nursing staff at the care home did not carry out physical observations appropriately for Rachel while back at home and did not document these appropriately, therefore being able to show a possible deterioration. A Chief Coroner's report following the incident also raised concerns about this nursing conduct not being fully investigated or reported to the NMC. The coroner concluded that had appropriate medical assistance been sought when Rachel's medical condition began to deteriorate she would have likely survived.

As part of the agenda to address the health inequalities of people with learning disabilities, the organisation Mencap established a referral system known as 'Rachel's Voice'.

Consider Rachel when reading chapters that include the following:

- Health inequalities
- Learning from lives and deaths of people with a learning disability and autistic people (LeDeR): National LeDeR Programme
- Diagnostic overshadowing
- Mental Capacity Act (2005)
- Safeguarding and whistleblowing in Transforming Care and mental health support for people with a learning disability
- Nursing observations

Thomas Rawnsley

In the early hours of 2 February 2015, Thomas Rawnsley suffered a cardiac arrest brought upon by a chest infection and tragically died two days later in hospital. Thomas was 20 years old, with Down syndrome, and had been residing in a care home since 2014 where he was placed by the Court of Protection following being detained under the Mental Health Act in an Assessment and Treatment unit. The unit could not meet Thomas's needs, being described as unable to cope with his behaviour, and the care home was an interim measure while a more suitable place could be found nearer to his family.

Thomas was placed at Kingdom House care home in Sheffield. Following Thomas's death his family told an inquest that they had often expressed concern about the care he was receiving there but that nothing had ever been done to address those concerns. The family reported concerns relating to Thomas's physical and mental well-being, saying that if Thomas ever reported feeling unwell this would be dismissed by staff as 'attention-seeking' behaviour. Thomas had limited verbal communication but did use some Makaton. It has also been reported that the staff were not well-trained and had limited experience in supporting people with learning disabilities and complex needs.

There are well-documented failings of care home staff, paramedic staff and medical staff in the days and hours leading up to Thomas's death. These include inadequate medical advice, poor health assessment and signs of deterioration through changes in behaviour and physical presentation being missed. Despite this the inquest found that Thomas died of natural causes and that engaging Article 2 of the European Convention on Human Rights was not appropriate. Using this would have meant acknowledging neglect which would or could have contributed to the death.

Consider Thomas when reading chapters that include the following:

- National LeDeR programme
- Health inequalities
- Communication
- The deteriorating patient
- Multi-disciplinary working and coordination of care
- Nursing observations

Laura Booth

Laura was admitted to Sheffield Hallamshire hospital at the age of 21 in 2016 for a routine eye operation. Laura had physical and learning disabilities. She had Partial Trisomy 13, which is a life-limiting genetic condition. Laura had limited verbal communication but would communicate using non-verbal methods and also used some Makaton. When Laura was admitted to hospital her parents were with her the whole time she was there until she died 24 days later due to malnutrition brought about by inadequate nutrition. The coroner identified that Laura's death was contributed to by neglect.

While in hospital, although Laura's parents noticed and reported that she was not eating and drinking adequately, they felt they were not listened to and nutritional assessment and monitoring, including charts to monitor her intake, were not implemented during her stay in hospital. The family maintain that all attempts made by Laura to communicate with medical and nursing staff were ignored.

The inquest into Laura's death also found that at no point had a Best Interests meeting taken place and that her care was not in accordance with the requirements of the Mental Capacity Act (2005) therefore making it unlawful.

Consider Laura when reading chapters that include the following:

- Best Interests and Mental Capacity Act (2005)
- Communication
- Nursing observations and the deteriorating patient
- National LeDeR Programme
- Inclusive communication: Creating positive outcomes – a mothers lived experience
- A reflection on communication and the use of hospital; passports within an acute hospital setting

The power of words

Why terminology is important

Andrea Page, Samantha Salmon and Helen Jones, with a contribution from Emmie Jeffrey

Why is this chapter important?

Language and how we refer to things changes and evolves constantly, as a result of different cultures interacting, advances in technology, new inventions and old words acquiring new meanings. Terminology is a collection of words that have a special meaning in any given subject.

The importance of choosing the right words can make all the difference in how we communicate effectively and how we value others.

Learning disability

The most current definition of learning disability is:

- a significantly reduced ability to understand new or complex information or to learn new skills (in other words people with a learning disability tend to take longer to learn and may need support to develop new skills, understand complicated information and interact with other people)

- a reduced ability to cope independently (in other words looking after themselves or living alone)

- has its onset before adulthood

- with a lasting effect on development

(Department of Health, 2001; NHS, 2022)

A person with a **learning disability** is someone who, from childhood, has had difficulty in learning and processing information so that it significantly reduces their ability to carry out the full range of everyday tasks. People with a learning disability are a very diverse group with a wide range of abilities. A learning disability can be identified through a combination of intelligence tests and measures of 'adaptive

DOI: 10.4324/9781003341765-3

behaviour' (i.e. a person's ability to carry out everyday tasks). In the UK the threshold for learning disability is set at an IQ of below 70. However, people with a learning disability do not fall into discrete groups, and IQ scores may not reflect how well they cope with life, nor are their abilities fixed forever (Cumella, 2015).

A **profound and multiple learning disability** is often viewed as a description rather than a clinical diagnosis. Some of you may have heard of the Weschler Adult Intelligence Scale (WAIS) which was used to guide policy and services. Whilst there are no definitive characteristics for a profound and multiple learning disability, there will be more than one disability and often co-morbidities in terms of health. Other additional disabling conditions include physical disabilities, sensory impairments, sensory processing difficulties, complex health needs (epilepsy, respiratory problems, dysphagia, eating and drinking problems), challenging behaviours (also known as behaviours of concern), mental health difficulties and self-injurious behaviour being common (Dalby & Knifton, 2012). Difficulties with communication are also common and about 80% of this group have physical impairments that affect their mobility. It is recognised that an individual with a profound and multiple learning disability will need maximum assistance and 24-hour support in all aspects of daily living (Doukas et al., 2017).

What do we mean by terminology?

Nurses use terminology to communicate effectively with one another, to communicate effectively with other health professionals and to communicate effectively with the people we are caring for, which includes their family and other carers. It is important to remember that terminology also provides judgement and can be loaded with negative connotations which is why this chapter focuses on words used to describe people with a learning disability.

Learning disability nursing has been shaped by different factors and societal norms: up to the 1940s the predominant term was 'mental deficiency', up to the 1970s the predominant term was 'mental subnormality', then it became 'mental handicap' and the current term used in the UK since 1991 is 'learning disability' or 'learning disabilities'. More recently the use of 'intellectual disabilities' across the UK has become more common (Mansell, 2010).

'Patients', who lived in institutions, became 'residents', 'clients', 'service users' as institutions closed and people moved into a variety of community care settings. Many are now viewed as 'tenants' or even 'citizens', who are renting and living in their own homes.

These changes around terminology came about because of societal changes in the language used to describe people, because of a positive change in values and attitudes, where we started listening to people. Language and attitudes have evolved to become more respectful towards people with disability and other minority groups in society and this is now reflected in the terminology we use and are comfortable with. Some changes are more subtle in nature and can be more difficult to adopt, in spite of our well-meaning values and intentions. However, it is important to reflect on our use of language and terminology in order for people to become more accepted and integrated within society.

TOP TIP

Listen carefully and change your language where you can. Think of the term 'respite' which is now defined as 'short breaks' and consider the quote below:

"Being told that we would probably need respite from our son when he reached his teens was not only a brutal statement in that moment, but also (temporarily) erased the joy, love, brilliance, knowledge, generosity and thoughtfulness that Connor would contribute to our family".

(Ryan, 2020, p. 65)

What is the issue?

Vocabulary, language and the terms used to refer to people with a learning disability may add to the discrimination they face, limitations on their human rights and the perception about their ability (Kassah, 2000; McClimens and Richardson, 2010). The terminology we use to refer to people with a learning disability often includes labels which would be the clinical language of the day and we need to be mindful of disability labels which may be associated with deficit, a person requiring rehabilitation and failure (Goodley, 2018). Orme wrote in 2003 that we live in a more 'politically correct' age and that this kind of labelling is part of nursing past, not our present or future. Orme emphasises that the way we describe people is usually a great indicator of the way we relate to them and in turn the way we treat them. The many incidences of abuse still reported and a recent Care Quality Commission (CQC) publication 'Experiences of being in hospital for people with a learning disability and autistic people' (2022) shows that people with a learning disability and autistic people are not getting the care they need, when they need it. McClimens and Richardson (2010) summarise the issue that people with a learning disability are trying to get by in their daily lives much like the rest of society. Given that perceptions about people with a learning disability are influenced by terminology, stigmatising language and labels can negatively impact on this aspiration (Andrews et al., 2019).

There can also be a confusion with the term learning difficulty or difficulties. Beardon (2017) and PHE (2018) state that a learning difficulty does not relate to intellectual disability at all, but to learning (in other words dyslexia or dyspraxia). A learning disability therefore, needs to be viewed as a 'complex way of being' (Gates 2001, cited in PHE 2018). Remember that no two people are alike.

Referring to individuals as 'a person *with* challenging behaviour' or 'this person *has* challenging behaviour' is also problematic, as that also suggests a diagnosis and therefore can lead to stigmatisation and exclusion from services. Challenging behaviour is simply how we talk about a range of behaviours that some people may display when their needs are not being met (The Challenging Behaviour Foundation). The term 'challenging behaviour' being misused in this way can lead to children and adults being denied the right to live an ordinary life in their local communities. The term 'challenging behaviour' should be used in its original sense to encourage carers and professionals to find effective ways of understanding the person's behaviour and underlying causes for this person to receive appropriate support.

As authors of this book, learning disability nurses and learning disability lecturers we read and hear learning disability or person with learning disabilities being repeatedly shortened to LD or PWLD and yet we have never seen or heard adult, children's, or mental health nursing shortened for example. Within professional discourse is it really such an inconvenience to type a few more letters or say learning disability in your written and spoken communications? We would like you to consider that the repeated use of acronyms to describe people with a learning disability is not using valuing language and not person centred, because language choices have social, cognitive and emotional significance (Andrews et al., 2019). The physical act of writing and saying the words in full reminds us all that the individual is a person first and not a label and therefore we should be saying or writing person with a learning disability/people with a learning disability; person with a profound and multiple learning disability/people with a profound and multiple learning disability.

What is important for people with a learning disability and how are 'we' doing with this (reflection by Emmie Jeffrey, first-year Learning Disability student nurse at Birmingham City University (BCU))

It is important to remember that behind the diagnosis of a learning disability, there is an individual human being with likes, dislikes, goals, aspirations, families and needs. There are a variety of things that differentiate those living with learning disability from others, as is the case for any other person. The learning disability is merely just another unique part of the individual's make-up. Having a learning disability may mean the person requires a level of support or they may have communication needs; however, it is not a label that they should be defined by.

I agree that terminology can impact on a person's wellbeing and opportunities, particularly in the example of 'challenging behaviour'. When a person displays challenging behaviour, they are perceived as 'violent' or 'difficult', when in reality they may be trying to communicate that they are lonely or ill. It is often forgotten that behaviour is used as another form of communication, which leads to the need to 'fix' the behaviour rather than understand what is causing the person to act this way. Being labelled as 'challenging' would be very degrading and distressing for someone who is already struggling to communicate their feelings.

I find the LD abbreviation interesting, as I had never considered that we do not use the same abbreviations for other nursing fields. I agree that this may become yet another label for people with learning disabilities to deal with.

It is clear that we have come a long way throughout the years with regard to terminology and I feel that by recognising the stigma surrounding the labels and abbreviations placed upon people we are promoting a much improved, person-centred way of supporting people.

I found the Public Health England (PHE) (2018) Learning Disabilities: Applying All Our Health webpage to be very informative, with a lot of statistics that bring home the importance of the support that learning disability nurses provide. The section on institutional discrimination was particularly interesting and relative to this chapter.

I am yet to attend placement with BCU, but I have worked for a number of years as a support worker with adults with learning disabilities. It is a sad truth that I have experienced brilliant individuals tied down by labels such as 'the autistic one'. It is only with knowledge, guidance and discussions such as those in this chapter that people will begin to understand how detrimental these labels can be to a person's wellbeing.

Useful links and resources

BILD: www.bild.org.uk and www.bris.ac.uk/cipold

Public Health England (PHE) (2018) Learning Disabilities: Applying All Our Health https://www.gov.uk/government/publications/learning-disability-applying-all-our-health/learning-disabilities-applying-all-our-health (accessed 13.12.2022)

The Challenging Behaviour Foundation   https://www.challengingbehaviour.org.uk/ (accessed 13.12.2022)

University of Hertfordshire, Intellectual Disability Policy in England. Available at: https://www.intellectualdisability.info/historic-articles/articles/intellectual-disability-policy-in-england (accessed 13.12.2022)

References

Andrews, E.E., Forber-Pratt, A.J., Mona, L.R., Lund, E.M., Pilarski, C.R. & Balter, R. (2019) #SaytheWord: a disability culture commentary on the erasure of 'disability'. *Rehabilitation Psychology*, 64(2): 111–118. doi: 10.1037/rep0000258. Epub 2019 Feb 14. PMID: 30762412.

Beardon, L. (2017) *Autism and Asperger Syndrome in Adults (overcoming common problems)*. London: Sheldon Press

Care Quality Commission (CQC) (2022) Experiences of being in hospital for people with a learning disability and autistic people. https://www.cqc.org.uk/publication/experiences-being-hospital-people-learning-disability-and-autistic-people/report?fbclid=IwAR0hu h18u3a8Gg0lYCYUgxRnInV-FpRG4Ps6t0DPY4jUzZ-6TIr3m5kmRDQ#mcgowan (accessed 8.11.2022)

Cumella, S. (2015) Shared-life communities: a review of research, conference paper. https://www.researchgate.net/publication/281714887_Shared-life_communities_a_review_of_research (accessed 8.11.2022)

Dalby, D. & Knifton, C. (2012) *Learning Disability Nurse Survival Guide: Common questions and answers for the learning disability nurse*. London: Quay Books.

Department of Health (2001) Valuing People – a New Strategy for Learning Disability for the 21st Century. Available at: https://www.gov.uk/government/publications/valuing-people-a-new-strategy-for-learning-disability-for-the-21st-century

Doukas, T., Fergusson, A., Fullerton, M. & Grace, J. (2017) Supporting people with profound and multiple learning disabilities: core and essential service standards. Available at: https://www.pmldlink.org.uk/wp-content/uploads/2017/11/Standards-PMLD-h-web.pdf

Gates, B. (2001) Valuing people: long awaited strategy for people with learning disabilities for the 21st Century in England, UK. *Journal of Learning Disabilities*, 5(3): 203–207.

Goodley, D. (2018) Understanding disability: biopsychology, biopolitics, and an in-between-all politics. *Adapted Physical Activity Quarterly*, 35: 308–319.

Grant, G., Ramcharan, P., Flynn, M. & Richardson, M. (eds) (2010) *Learning Disability: A Life Cycle Approach*, 2nd edition. Maidenhead: Open University Press/McGraw-Hill Education.

Kassah, A. K. (2000) Terminology – from language to action. *Disability and Rehabilitation*, 22(11): 515–518.

Mansell, J. (2010) Raising our sights: services for adults with profound intellectual and multiple disabilities. *Tizard Learning Disability Review*, 15(3): 5–12. https://doi.org/10.5042/tldr.2010.0399

McClimens, A. & Richardson, M. (2010) in Grant, G., Ramcharan, P., Flynn, M. & Richardson, M. (eds), *Learning Disability: A Life Cycle Approach*, 2nd edition. Maidenhead: Open University Press/McGraw-Hill Education.

NHS (2022) Overview of learning disabilities. Available at: https://www.nhs.uk/conditions/learning-disabilities/ (accessed 13.12.2022)

Orme, E. (2003) A rose by any other name. *Learning Disability Practice*, 6(9): 18–20.

Public Health England (PHE) (2018) *Learning Disabilities: Applying All Our Health* https://www.gov.uk/government/publications/learning-disability-applying-all-our-health/learning-disabilities-applying-all-our-health (accessed 13.12.2022)

Ryan, S. (2020) *Love, Learning Disabilities and Pockets of Brilliance: How Practitioners Can Make a Difference to the Lives of Children, Families and adults*. London: Jessica Kingsley.

3

The Learning Disability nursing student and apprentice voice

Samantha Salmon, Christine Cooper, Jamie White, Blessing Taiwo and Jemima Tandoh

Why is it important that student nurses and apprentices from the four fields of nursing (learning disability, adult, children's and mental health) receive their theoretical learning together?

> Studying together with other cohort nursing students puts us in a position of gaining knowledge and skills of each other's field of nursing as we will all come across patients presenting with any condition… This also will help bridge the gap of health inequalities experienced by people with learning disabilities.
>
> (Jemima Tandoh)

Through reflective discussions, learning disability nursing students and apprentices highlighted that receiving their theoretical learning together not only empowered those from other fields to better meet the needs of people with a learning disability within their scope of practice but also increased awareness of the learning disability nursing profession and career opportunities for students from other fields of nursing. One student reflected on the potential for further study and commented on students from other fields who had expressed interest in becoming dual-qualified following shared learning. They highlighted the importance of breaking myths, overcoming barriers and fears for learners who had little confidence, knowledge or experience of learning disability and identified the *unlearning* that needed to take place for students who had arrived in higher education with at best incorrect and at worst negative preconceptions.

What are your experiences of other people's perceptions of learning disability and learning disability nursing?

The group reflected on when *they* first became aware of what a learning disability was. Some shared their experiences of times with family members who had a diagnosis of learning disability and others did not have the opportunity to interact with

DOI: 10.4324/9781003341765-4

a person with a learning disability until later in life. It was felt that there is not much knowledge or awareness of learning disability nursing as a career within the general public and learning disability students stated that they had not found out about this career option until shortly before applying for the course, despite having personal or professional experience in supporting people with a learning disability. By reflecting on their own knowledge and experiences this led to empathy for the misconceptions of others and all reported that they had experienced a misunderstanding of what a learning disability is and the role and value of a learning disability nurse. In addition to other professionals not knowing what a learning disability nurse does, some also voiced that they did not realise learning disability nurses had the same level of training, skills and clinical expertise as other fields of nursing, which had led to the misconception that learning disability nurses are not 'real' nurses. Paradoxically, examples were shared where recognition of the expertise of learning disability nurses was demonstrated; however, this seemed to result in deferral and referral of the needs of people with a learning disability. There was a sense of other healthcare professionals feeling that they did not need to know about how to meet the needs of a person with a learning disability as the specialist learning disability nurse would do this for them. On the surface, this could seem understandable and whilst no professional can, or should be expected to, know everything this is discriminatory and the first step of the 'othering' of people with a learning disability. We discussed the Mencap Death by Indifference reports (Mencap 2007, 2012) where it was identified that avoidable deaths had occurred through institutional discrimination across a variety of health and social care services; it was described as a 'national disgrace' in 2007.

> It would be better if others realised that often it doesn't have to be complicated or something to be feared, reasonable adjustments are something that any professional can put in place.
>
> (Christine Cooper)

Can you outline a positive experience you have had in relation to the care of people with a learning disability?

As a group, we reflected on advocating for and involving the person and role modelling how to do this when educating peers and other professionals. The importance of acknowledging and identifying where a person has a learning disability, reducing the risk of diagnostic overshadowing and the need for better application of trauma-informed care across a range of health and social care settings was evident through these discussions. Whilst specific details have been omitted to maintain confidentiality the examples below were felt to be broad enough to help contextualise these areas.

When discussing the instances where people had experienced multiple traumatic life events it was found that there were occasions where this had not been fully considered when professionals were reviewing care. We talked about how impactful a single traumatic life event can be for a person, let alone several, yet many people with a learning disability are at increased risk of experiencing these or facing additional barriers to accessing the right support following such events. Often all it took was for one person to voice this to a room of professionals and really listen to the individual to find what was causing them the most distress and making that necessary change. In the examples given, it was a common finding that seemingly small, and often common-sense, observations resulted in other professionals making the needed reasonable adjustments to reduce distress and meet the person's holistic needs.

Another example from within a mental health setting highlighted how important it was to recognise when a person has a learning disability as not all people will have a diagnosis and many have fallen through gaps in the system. In this case a learning disability student queried whether an individual may have undiagnosed autism and/or a learning disability and highlighted that the likelihood of experiencing problems with mental health are reportedly higher. This observation led to a referral to the community learning disability team resulting in more professionals being included at the next multidisciplinary meeting – they had to get a bigger room! Following this additional input the individual's plan of care was amended with extra consideration of the impact of disturbances of their routine and preferences and amendments to the environment and communication of staff.

Although there were many more examples of the positive differences student nurses and apprentices had made to the care of people with a learning disability in practice these have been included as they were felt to relate most to the case studies outlined in this section.

Can you outline one positive experience in relation to teaching and learning at university where there was collaboration and shared learning about caring for people with a learning disability across fields?

This was initially discussed in relation to sessions where learning disability students shared their knowledge and expertise in certain areas, such as mental capacity and communication when educating other fields of nursing in the classroom. One specific example a student shared was in regards to a lecture about epilepsy:

> Even though it initially started out as an epilepsy session it evolved to educate a lot of students about how to support people with a learning disability too. As students from the learning disability field of nursing had had a lot of experience in supporting people with a learning disability who also had epilepsy we were able to share our experiences and show our knowledge which felt good.
>
> (Jamie White)

Students also shared how they liked the interactive taught sessions where they were put into groups with students from other fields and had the opportunity to talk about differences and similarities across fields, sharing ideas and their experiences across different placement settings. They remembered role-play sessions and mock environments and situations which initially pushed them out of their comfort zones but felt that the subjects and topics 'came alive' and they valued the learning from others.

One student reflected on the crossing over of fields when supporting a child with a learning disability and how they had benefitted from the knowledge and skills of a nursing student from another field in their first year:

> I only knew about utilising communication skills like pictures, visual aids, storytelling techniques and videos when caring for someone with learning disabilities until a student from another nursing field in the group suggested role playing using a teddy bear to demonstrate medical intervention to a child with learning disabilities.
>
> (Jemima Tandoh)

Another peer built upon this and reflected on what they recalled as the most powerful teaching session that they had; this was delivered by a mother of a child with a learning disability discussing their personal experience of univentricular heart transplant and how powerful this was:

> Having the opportunity to hear a real experience and the opportunity to ask questions and reflect on … and his family's journey was such a creative way to bring our learning to life. I do not think that any student hearing this will forget it and so the benefits of this impacting future care are so valuable.
>
> (Christine Cooper)

They shared their belief of the benefits of creative teaching techniques that allow space for students from all fields of nursing by promoting discussion where learners' own experiences could then enhance that learning further.

References

Mencap (2007) *Death by Indifference: Following the Treat Me Right! Report.* London: Mencap. Available at: https://www.mencap.org.uk/sites/default/files/2016-06/DBIreport.pdf

Mencap (2012) *Death by Indifference: 74 Deaths and Counting.* Mencap: London. Available at: https://www.mencap.org.uk/sites/default/files/2016-08/Death%20by%20 Indifference%20-%2074%20deaths%20and%20counting.pdf

4

About me and how I became Chief Executive of All Wales People First

Joe Powell

My name is Joe Powell, and I was diagnosed with Asperger Syndrome at the age of 20 in 1996. At that time, I had many mental health issues (depression and anxiety) and had made attempts at suicide and had incidents of self-harm. I was non-verbal/ selective mute for the best part of 11 years. I believe this was a post-traumatic stress disorder (PTSD) response to years of being misunderstood as a person with autism. Prior to this I struggled with the work in school and was mocked for being behind the other children. I became the class clown to cover up my shortfalls and I got into a lot of trouble in school because of it. At home too I was very difficult for my parents to manage. My behaviour deteriorated and I was suspended from school on two occasions. When I was 15 years old, I changed schools at the recommendation of a child psychologist who assessed me. Because I didn't know anyone in the new school I knuckled down and worked, and for the first time was seen in a very positive light. My parents were thrilled, and I became a model student. I was praised for being such a lovely quiet lad. This became an obsession, in which I eventually stopped speaking at all. I liken it to anorexia but instead of starving myself of food, I starved myself of words. If I spoke or ever felt I let my high standards slip I got really distressed and needed very lengthy and complex reassurances to alleviate my anxiety. This put an enormous strain on the family unit.

When diagnosed with Asperger Syndrome, my parents and I thought sending me to an autism care service to be 'fixed up' would make me 'normal' and able to live in the real world like my peers. Our expectations were wholly unrealistic. My first care service in Manchester did not work. One of the reasons for this was because my mental health issues and trauma were so severe that it was not possible for the service to work with me. They were also not geared up in my opinion to help people with autism to move on to a more independent life (although some did). Also, the environment I was in was more conducive to people with autism and learning disabilities who had profound care needs. My issues were largely mental health issues. I was very obsessive and an incredible perfectionist and was very competitive because of it. I had to be the 'most' at everything. Even the most autistic

DOI: 10.4324/9781003341765-5

person. I believe the latter was because of the trauma I suffered through living with a so-called 'hidden disability' which meant I was misunderstood and vulnerable and did not want to be in that situation ever again.

The care home environment I was in was highly toxic. I did not understand the distress behaviours displayed by the others using the service and I judged them on that behaviour. I intervened to protect the staff (initially) when they were under attack thinking I was defending them. In the end my own distress behaviour became more and more frequent. This was because one service user used to display aggressive and loud behaviour for days on end and attacking him was the only way to stop it (temporarily) and give me some relief for a couple of days, before the cycle began again. This got me into trouble and challenged my delusion of being perfect, which began when I was 15. I had an enormous mental health crisis and my wellbeing deteriorated after that point. I stopped cleaning myself and spent all my time sleeping. The service thought I was being lazy and not trying. My parents believed that I was getting 'worse' rather than 'better' when in this service. One day I drank some cleaning fluid and was rushed to the local hospital. My parents were really concerned for my wellbeing at that stage. On leaving the service I eventually gained access to my files and was horrified to discover that my behaviours were attributed to me wanting to intimidate other people. None of the details of my living circumstances were recorded.

I moved to a new care service in Newport, South Wales in 2002 to be closer to my parents. My dad's department had moved from Gateshead in the North East of England to Glascoed in South Wales. We thought a new service and having family close by would give me the chance to make a new start. My new start was interesting. The idea was that in my new service I would change from being the 'least able' service user to the 'most able' service user to reverse the trend from my last service. Although it was intended to be a positive spin and a positive philosophy for my new start in life, it really felt that I was being given a second chance and that this second chance was dependent on my 'good behaviour'. Indeed, I had to sign a contract of good behaviour as part of starting my new service. It meant that any distress behaviour would not be tolerated, and I was expected to be less dependent than before. This was difficult if not impossible at times. I was highly anxious and highly sensitive and went from having intense reassurance in my service in Manchester to none overnight. It felt really cruel at the time and I believed the approach taken by some staff amounted to bullying. One day after being intensely polite for some time despite what I considered to be bullying behaviour from some staff, I snapped at the house manager telling her I was not happy with how I was being treated and I stormed out of the house. The overall service manager was summoned to deal with me the next day and he asked me very sternly if I 'wanted a new service' without making any attempt to ascertain the facts about what had happened. I took this as a threat, and I knew that I could not go to them if I had any problems in the future.

However, over time, by getting into a routine with my day centre and pushing myself to be more outgoing, I made a lot of progress, was very popular with the other service users and became what I called their 'pet autistic'. The one whose progress would be used to show what a good service they were. The reality was that I put in a sink-or-swim situation, and I swum, with a lot of help in the background from my parents. I faked it till I made it as they say in terms of my outward facade and demeanour, but it was not real and covered up the long-term social anxieties and mental health problems which were not addressed. This included my difficulties with assertiveness and the mental health difficulties that caused me to be non-verbal. It was difficult for me to be a 'service user' because the regime was not appropriate for me. The regime felt very school-like, and it was difficult for someone like me to accept some of the patronising and bullying behaviour from some support staff. Staff who frankly didn't even know what my needs were.

After two years of making positive progress, it was time to move on, but my service would not let this happen. They said if I left the care system, I would be sectioned in three months. I hit another mental health crisis. I approached an independent advocate who told my local authorities about my situation, and they contacted a support broker to work with me on an individual budget. That was the turning point. An individual budget meant that I employed my own staff team and lived independently in my own flat in the community. I went from a care service costing £130,000 to an individual budget costing £28,000 and had more support than I had ever had before. Within two years the difference in me and the progress I made was dramatic. Year after year I gave more and more money back to my local authority (unspent) and my budget was reduced. Eventually I needed no support at all and now live completely independently. The difference I believe came about because the approach to supporting me shifted from focusing on the things I struggled with to building on the things I was good at. My individual budget focused on the things I needed for a good life.

In 2012 an advertisement for a 'National Director' for All Wales People First was shown to me by a lady called Julie Tucker of WECIL, an organisation that used to review my individual budget. All Wales People First were looking for someone with lived experience of learning disability services to head the organisation. I applied and I got the job and have been here ever since. My role was rebranded to Chief Executive because of the extra responsibilities that I have taken on. My life has changed beyond recognition now. I gained a degree, live completely independently and have no support whatsoever. All because a different approach was taken. I believe that many other people with autism and learning disabilities could be living much better lives than they currently do if they were supported with the same philosophy. All Wales People First is a national umbrella body for self-advocacy groups for people with learning disabilities in Wales. We believe that self-advocacy is the most important form of advocacy. We want to bring about real change for our members so that they can be active and contributing citizens. I want to use the opportunity that All Wales People First has given me to bring about that change.

What are your thoughts about low arousal as an approach?

As an approach I would say it is essential. I believe it is the way to bridge that gap between people with autism/learning disabilities (often under significant stress and with limited communication capacity) and those who are neurotypical who traditionally support them. It is also critical when supporting people who often experience sensory issues. This is not only to do with the five senses; in my experience language and tone of voice can cause distress if not understood. Low arousal should be preventative and not just reactive and must therefore be a constant, not just a technique we pull out of the bag when someone is in a crisis.

I would also say that as part of a preventative rather than a reactive approach it is important that we don't unintentionally create a culture of high arousal through only responding to those in crisis. I have seen situations in which staff don't understand a person is struggling until they show distress behaviour. It is important we recognise when someone is struggling and support them at the earliest opportunity. That we know the subtle signs not just the obvious ones. That can only happen by understanding the needs of the person you are supporting.

For the low-arousal approach to work I believe we must ensure a work culture exists of reflection and humility, where staff are encouraged to reflect without fear of judgement and to take constructive criticism. I believe gearing up staff to be ready for a culture that enables this should be the starting point and the first thing new staff are trained in. However, even the best-quality training is of little use unless the person being trained chooses to embrace it and feels passionate about their role. We need the right people with the right values.

Are you aware of any organisations who introduced low arousal for people with learning disabilities and/or autism?

I am aware of organisations that say they are low arousal and champion the concept of low arousal, but I am not sure whether they do it in practice. I worry that low arousal, like 'person centred', may be a concept that many buy into in principle but don't fully understand it in practice. The care situations I have lived in, for instance, may focus on low arousal in terms of some of the environmental changes they may make to a service but not understand the impact that their own behaviour can have on others. Even some people who champion the low-arousal approach can be unintentionally highly obnoxious and completely unaware of it.

For instance, when I moved into my second residential care service, I could see the staff looking at me outside of my flat through the kitchen window, whispering to each other like I was a poisoned insect. It felt like they were weighing up the 'retard'. I felt this deeply and it impacted on my mood. It also made me feel like I was not wanted in the service, and that they felt vulnerable and out of their depth in working with me. Many people may think that I am the exception rather than the rule because I can read those signs, but I disagree. I believe that people, even with profound learning disabilities, still subconsciously absorb these vibes. I believe it is a primal human instinct and is picked up by the subconscious. If a person feels those around them are judging them or are not confident in supporting them then it is bound to make them feel vulnerable and heighten their anxieties. If you are a person who is limited in the way they can express their emotions the pent-up frustration has to be released somehow. This results in distress behaviours and ironically, if misunderstood further fuels the fear of those supporting them.

I do wonder sometimes if this was one of the reasons for the poor treatment of people with learning disabilities in high-profile cases such as Winterbourne View. Poorly trained staff feel threatened and entitled to 'settle the score'. There is a world of difference between bad behaviour and distress behaviour even if sometimes they look the same. In my wider experience as a user of services in the care sector, staff would be trained on autism or low-arousal approaches but still refer to the people they were supporting as 'kicking off' and feeling a sense of frustration that they were not able to exercise some form of retribution. It is important to remember that football hooligans 'kick off' while people with learning disabilities do not.

What has been the impact on people's lives?

I really believe the impact, if done correctly, is everything. The impact on the wellbeing of the person being supported and their quality of life is no doubt enhanced, incidents of distress behaviours will be reduced and we win the trust of the person we are supporting. If we win the trust of the person we are supporting, then we are much more likely to be able to make further progress in their personal development (teaching new life and independent skills for instance). It also makes for a better working environment for the staff, and I would hope prevent burnout and stress. I believe so many problems are caused by the physical and working environments people with autism and learning disabilities are placed into and that this is still very misunderstood by many. This misunderstanding perpetuates a culture of deficit-centred thinking amongst practitioners as well as making their own jobs much harder.

Why do you think student nurses should learn about and use low-arousal techniques?

I believe there are two main reasons for this. I think, firstly, an understanding of low-arousal techniques would educate the nurses about the nature of distress behaviour and why it happens, and equip them to know how to best handle the situation. More importantly, it is key to building empathy for the person we are working with. If taken at face value, distress behaviour can be taken personally and, in some cases, make the nurse or practitioner feel threatened and take a dislike to the person they are working with. This may affect their approach and further exacerbate the situation. Once we are equipped to both understand why the behaviour is happening and what we can do to support the person we are working with we equip nurses to feel less frightened, more empowered and more effective as nurses when working with people who may be in distress. But most importantly of all, a low-arousal approach will prevent many of the unnecessary causes of anxiety and distress from happening in the first place.

5

Learning from lives and deaths of people with learning disability and autistic people

The national LeDeR programme in practice

Katie Meah

The LeDeR programme was established in May 2015, and was initially known as the Learning Disabilities Mortality Review (LeDeR) programme (Heslop et al., 2022). The acronym of LeDeR was created using the letters from the title of the programme – **Le**arning **D**isabiliti**e**s **R**eview. There have been a number of changes to the programme and in March 2021 the national LeDeR policy was revised, changing the programme name to Learning from lives and deaths: People with a learning disability and autistic people (NHSE, 2021). The LeDeR acronym continues to be used.

LeDeR is a service improvement programme which aims to:

- Improve care,
- Reduce health inequalities and
- Prevent early death of people with a learning disability and autistic people.

There is an overlap between these aims; if care is improved, this should reduce health inequalities which includes the premature mortality (early death) amongst people with learning disabilities and autistic people.

Improving care

People with learning disabilities, autistic people and their families often encounter lots of different services and professionals throughout their life; however, literature shows that people often experience poor care, and do not have their needs met (Emerson & Baines, 2011; Heslop et al., 2014; White et al., 2023).

DOI: 10.4324/9781003341765-6

Improving care for people with a learning disability and autistic people within the health and social care system requires a coordinated approach; this includes individual actions from practitioners as well as strategic leadership to ensure the delivery of high-quality consistent care.

Figure 5.1 shows some of the services and areas that make up the health and social care system. It highlights the breadth of services and practitioners involved in health and social care and the scale of the challenge in improving care consistently across an ever-changing health and social care system.

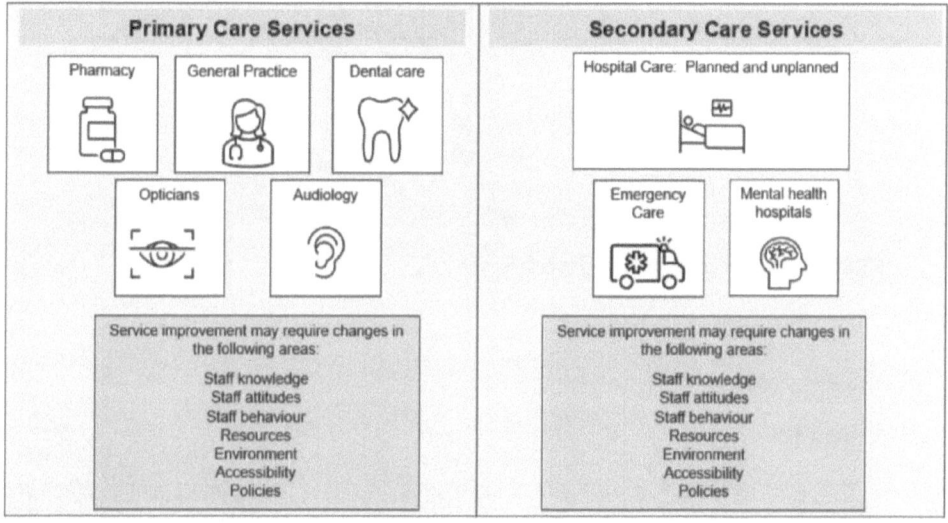

FIGURE 5.1A Services primary and secondary

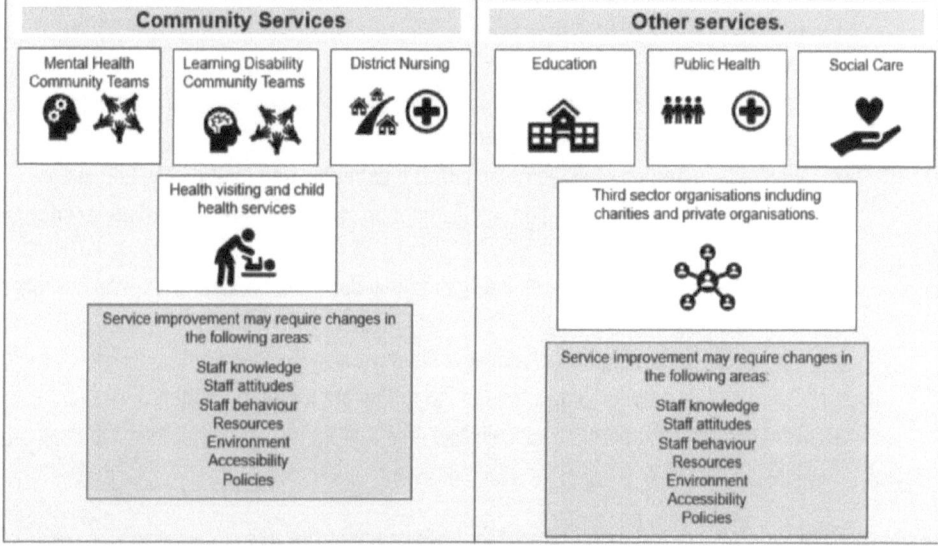

FIGURE 5.1B Services community and other

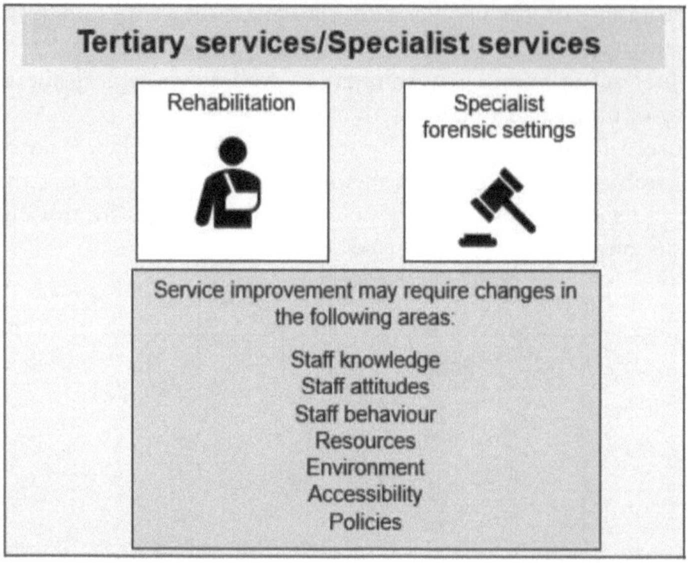

FIGURE 5.1C Services tertiary and specialist services

TOP TIP

It is important that you are aware of the different services that support people. When you are working with someone, it is important to know who else is involved, so that you can work together and coordinate care and ensure it is person centred.

How to improve services for people you are working with:

■ Smile and reassure people.

■ Listen to people.

■ Find out the way the person communicates and use this to help you understand the person and explain what is happening.

■ Find out if a person requires reasonable adjustments and make these happen.

■ Provide accessible information – this might be easier to read information, or information in a different format.

■ Use an interpreter if the person or their family does not speak English – do not rely on family members to interpret.

■ Find out about the person's health condition.

■ Talk to someone who knows the person to find out more about them.

■ Find out what the person is usually like – so that if there are differences you can report and act on these.

Thinking Point: What else can you do to improve services?

All these actions are achievable, and part of professional codes, policies and expectations; however, learning from LeDeR reports (White et al., 2022; White et al, 2023) shows that they are not always practised.

Reducing health inequalities

The King's Fund (2022) define health inequalities as 'avoidable, unfair and systematic differences in health between different groups of people'. Health inequalities can mean that some groups are more likely to experience poorer health, they may die sooner than others and they may not be able to access services to maintain or manage their health.

Sadly, we know that many people with learning disabilities experience multiple inequalities, which relate to poorer health outcomes, premature death and poor access to health services (Emerson & Baines, 2011; Williams et al., 2017; White et al., 2023). The LeDeR reviewers who work on the LeDeR programme gather information relating to a person's life and death, which includes health information and access to services. This information is analysed to identify inequalities and develop service improvement plans which address these inequalities.

There are lots of reasons why individuals may experience inequality. It may be related to a single aspect of a person's identity, for instance disability, gender, ethnicity, age, socioeconomic group or sexuality; there is a growing recognition that individuals with a learning disability and autistic people often have a number of these characteristics which intersect, meaning that people experience multiple disadvantage which compounds the inequalities (Hassiotis, 2020; Umpleby et al., 2023, White et al., 2023).

TOP TIP

Remember, equality is not treating everyone the same; it is ensuring that there is equal opportunity and access. Think about what you can do to promote equal opportunities and access wherever you are working.

Preventing early death of people with a learning disability and autistic people

Health inequalities can lead to premature death. Findings from the LeDeR programme have shown that people with learning disabilities die at an earlier age than people without learning disabilities.

Figure 5.2 shows the average age of death of people with learning disabilities whose death was reported to LeDeR between 2018 and 2022 (White et al., 2023).

The deaths of autistic people have been included in the LeDeR programme since March 2021; however, there is limited information to date about the specific needs of this group.

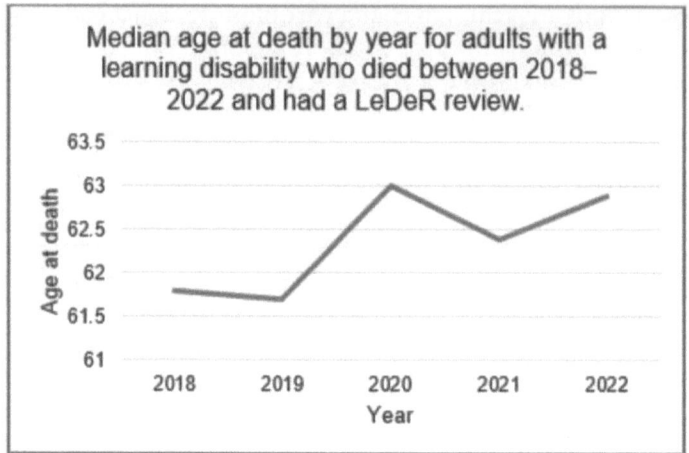

FIGURE 5.2 Graph showing median age of death

People with learning disabilities will experience the same health conditions as the general population; they may be overweight, constipated, have epilepsy and have mental health conditions. However, people with learning disabilities may be more likely to experience these, and paradoxically less likely to receive the care and treatment to manage or treat the condition (NHS Digital, 2023). Some of these conditions are more pertinent to people with learning disabilities and may even present differently and this will be discussed in more detail within Chapter 14, 'Conditions that all nurses and allied health professionals need to be aware of in people with learning disabilities'.

There are several reasons why people with a learning disability may be more likely to develop specific health conditions. One factor may be due to biological reasons; the evidence shows that there are syndromes where the person also has learning disabilities which are related to higher risk of some health conditions. For instance, people with Down syndrome are more likely to develop dementia, have thyroid dysfunction and coeliac disease (Rubin et al., 2016) whereas people with tuberous sclerosis are more likely to have epilepsy and kidney problems and lesions can develop in the lungs, on the skin or in the heart (Martin et al., 2017).

TOP TIP

If you are working with someone with a syndrome, there may be specific health conditions that are linked to the syndrome; include this information in their care plan or hospital passport so that people are aware.

Effective health care interventions and access to health services may be able to mitigate the impact of these conditions on the individual and may mean that they can be managed. For instance, if people with Down syndrome are regularly screened for signs of dementia, this may be detected at an earlier stage.

People with learning disabilities may experience diagnostic overshadowing. Diagnostic overshadowing is when a person's learning disability is used as a reason to explain a person's behaviour rather than considering any additional underlying health needs. This means that the person's needs may be unmet because the learning disability diagnosis overshadows everything else and will be at greater risk of deterioration of health or even death. (Public Health England, 2023).

TOP TIP

Always rule out a physical cause for any changes you observe in someone's behaviour. To do this ensure that you have accurate information about how a person displays pain and what their typical behaviour is; if you notice changes, write down your concerns, how long this has been happening and raise these with the wider care team – this might be the GP, psychiatrist, community team, or staff directly supporting the person.

The LeDeR programme began in 2015, led by Pauline Heslop and a team at Bristol University. During this time, there were pilot sites which were completing LeDeR reviews, and the methodology, resources and systems were being developed to ensure the programme was functional and could meet the aims of the programme. For a full overview of how the LeDeR programme was established and what a LeDeR review aims to do, see Heslop et al. (2022).

The aims of the original programme were:

- To support improvements in the quality of health and social care service delivery for people with learning disabilities.

- To help reduce premature mortality and health inequalities for people with learning disabilities.

June 2021 onwards

The first national LeDeR policy was published by NHS England in March 2021 and came into effect in June 2021 (NHSE, 2021). All Integrated Care Boards (ICBs) had duties and responsibilities as part of the programme to carry out LeDeR reviews of the deaths of people with learning disabilities and autistic people who were registered with a GP in their local area (NHSE, n.d)

Initial reviews and focused reviews were introduced

Focused reviews involve the reviewer gathering information from several sources and providing an in-depth summary of any health conditions. The comprehensive nature of the review means that a full understanding of the person's contacts with services and their experiences can be explored to identify areas for service improvement as well as any examples of positive practice.

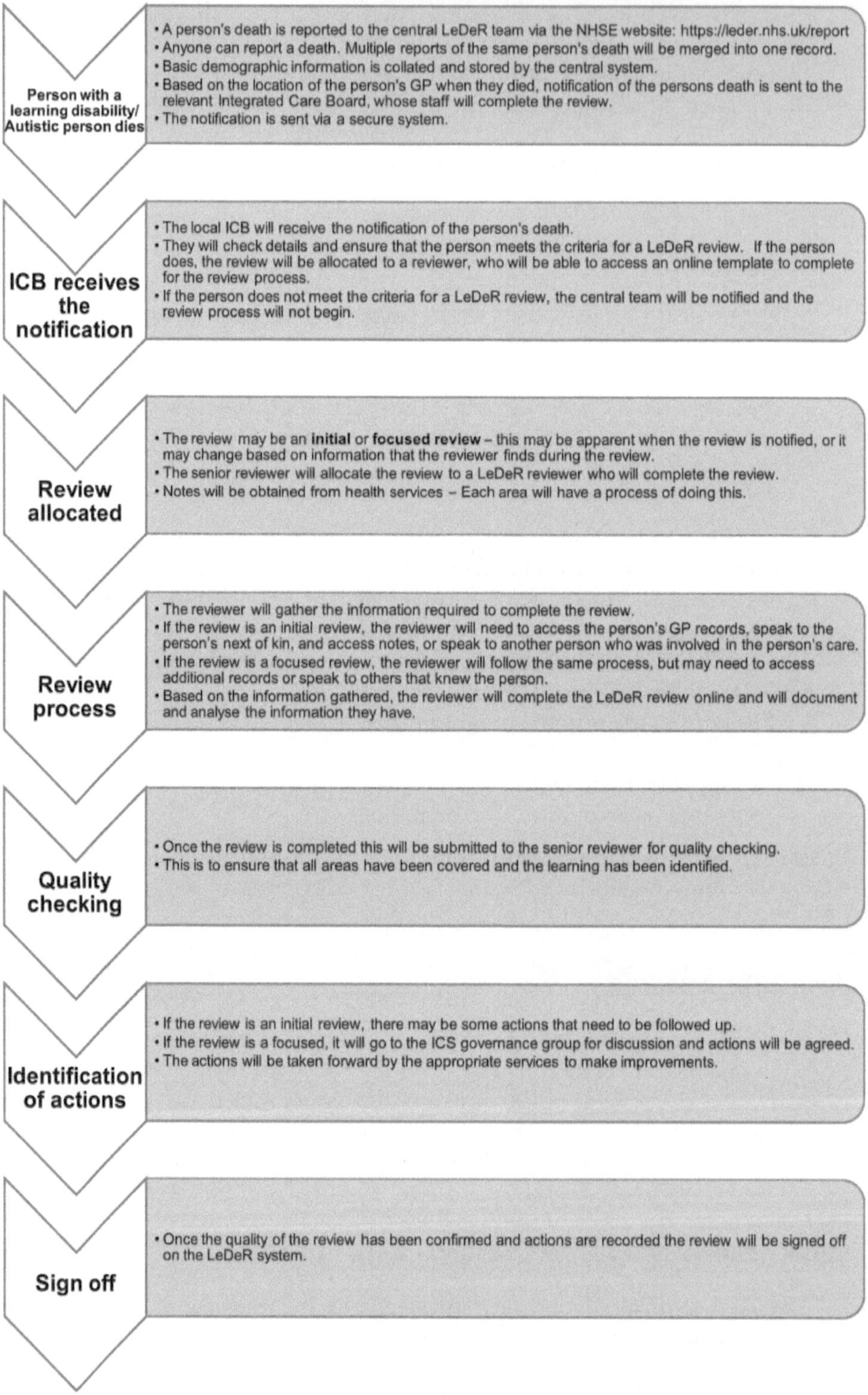

Person with a learning disability/Autistic person dies
- A person's death is reported to the central LeDeR team via the NHSE website: https://leder.nhs.uk/report
- Anyone can report a death. Multiple reports of the same person's death will be merged into one record.
- Basic demographic information is collated and stored by the central system.
- Based on the location of the person's GP when they died, notification of the persons death is sent to the relevant Integrated Care Board, whose staff will complete the review.
- The notification is sent via a secure system.

ICB receives the notification
- The local ICB will receive the notification of the person's death.
- They will check details and ensure that the person meets the criteria for a LeDeR review. If the person does, the review will be allocated to a reviewer, who will be able to access an online template to complete for the review process.
- If the person does not meet the criteria for a LeDeR review, the central team will be notified and the review process will not begin.

Review allocated
- The review may be an **initial** or **focused review** – this may be apparent when the review is notified, or it may change based on information that the reviewer finds during the review.
- The senior reviewer will allocate the review to a LeDeR reviewer who will complete the review.
- Notes will be obtained from health services – Each area will have a process of doing this.

Review process
- The reviewer will gather the information required to complete the review.
- If the review is an initial review, the reviewer will need to access the person's GP records, speak to the person's next of kin, and access notes, or speak to another person who was involved in the person's care.
- If the review is a focused review, the reviewer will follow the same process, but may need to access additional records or speak to others that knew the person.
- Based on the information gathered, the reviewer will complete the LeDeR review online and will document and analyse the information they have.

Quality checking
- Once the review is completed this will be submitted to the senior reviewer for quality checking.
- This is to ensure that all areas have been covered and the learning has been identified.

Identification of actions
- If the review is an initial review, there may be some actions that need to be followed up.
- If the review is a focused, it will go to the ICS governance group for discussion and actions will be agreed.
- The actions will be taken forward by the appropriate services to make improvements.

Sign off
- Once the quality of the review has been confirmed and actions are recorded the review will be signed off on the LeDeR system.

FIGURE 5.3 Review process diagram including focused and initial reviews

Initial reviews do not ask as many specific questions, and they are shorter reviews. They still require the reviewer to speak to the person's next of kin, look at GP records, speak to another professional who knew the person and answer some questions related to cause of death, advanced care planning and mental capacity.

A key difference between initial and focused reviews is the care grading; this is not completed for initial reviews. When reviewers complete focused reviews, they use their knowledge and judgement based on the information they have gathered to grade the quality of the care the person received and the availability and effectiveness of the care they received. The care grading is between 1 and 6; care graded at 1 or 2 indicates that the care fell short of good practice and contributed to the person's death. Care graded at 6 shows that there was evidence that the person received excellent care.

The care grading is contained in Figure 5.4.

LeDeR aims to highlight the positive practice that exists across organisations, so that this can be replicated and shared for local and national learning as well as identifying areas which need improvement.

The decision as to whether reviews are focused or initial depends on whether they meet the criteria for a focused review. Focused reviews take place if:

- The person's family requests a focused review, *or*

- The person who died is from a minority ethnic group.

People from minority ethnic groups who have a learning disability experience additional challenges in accessing healthcare and experience greater health inequalities, (Robertson et al., 2019; Salmi, 2023) and the data from the LeDeR annual reports show that there are fewer deaths reported to the programme than would be expected. The 'double discrimination' that people from ethnic minorities experience can be due to language barriers, a lack of cultural competence within services and a lack of access to specialist services (Umpleby, 2023).

Grade	Quality of care	Availability and effectiveness of services
6	This was excellent care (it exceeded expected good practice). Please identify in learning and recommendations what features of care made it excellent and consider how current practice could learn from this.	Availability and effectiveness of services was excellent and exceeded the expected standard.
5	This was good care (it met expected good practice). Please identify in the review learning and recommendations any features of care that current practice could learn from.	Availability and effectiveness of services was good and met the expected standard.
4	This was satisfactory care (it fell short of expected good practice in some areas but this did not significantly impact on the person's wellbeing). Please address these issues in your recommendations for service improvement, and identify in learning and recommendations any features of care that current practice could learn from.	Availability and effectiveness of services fell short of the expected standard in some areas but this did not significantly impact on the person's wellbeing.
3	Care fell short of expected good practice and this did impact on the person's wellbeing but did not contribute to the cause of death. Please address these issues in your recommendations for service improvement, and identify any features of care that current practice could learn from.	Availability and effectiveness of services fell short of the expected standard and this did impact on the person's wellbeing but did not contribute to the cause of death.
2	Care fell short of expected good practice and this significantly impacted on the person's wellbeing and/or had the potential to contribute to the cause of death.	Availability and effectiveness of services fell short of the expected standard and this significantly impacted on the person's wellbeing and/or had the potential to contribute to the cause of death.
1	Care fell far short of expected good practice and this contributed to the cause of death.	Availability and effectiveness of services fell far short of the expected standard and this contributed to the cause of death.

FIGURE 5.4 Overview of care grading

> **TOP TIP**
>
> Always be vigilant for discriminatory practice and unconscious bias. Work with individuals in a holistic way, showing respect for them and their culture.

LeDeR expanded to include reviewing deaths of people who were autistic without having a diagnosis of a learning disability

Evidence suggests autistic people experience poorer health than individuals without autism and are more likely to experience mental illness, epilepsy and cardiovascular conditions (Mason et al., 2019; O'Nions et al., 2024) in addition to barriers accessing health services; however, there has not been a systematic approach which looks at this issue in detail.

Learning disability and autism are very different diagnoses; however, it is anticipated that through the LeDeR programme there may be shared learning and opportunities for service improvement which will reduce inequalities for autistic people and people with learning disabilities (NHSE, 2021). The number of reviews reported is significantly less than what would be expected, given the estimated prevalence of autism is between 0.77 and 2.12% (O'Nions et al., 2023). Again, this does not mean that autistic people are not dying; it means that their deaths are not reported.

Learning from LeDeR

Local service improvement is a crucial element of LeDeR, and reviews can highlight areas of positive practice that can be shared and replicated across the integrated care system leading to improvements in services. LeDeR reviews can also provide a focus upon local services where processes and systems may not be working well, providing an opportunity to bring together stakeholders who can work together to make local change.

A focused review enables the reviewer to gather a large amount of information to fully understand the life and death of the person being reviewed and to raise any issues about the care received so that improvements can be made.

LeDeR is not an investigation, nor a complaint process. There are other processes which may take place before an LeDeR review if there are concerns raised – for instance a complaint, a coroner's inquest or a serious incident investigation. In these cases, an LeDeR review may need to wait until these processes are complete and the findings may inform the review.

Conclusion

The LeDeR programme developed because of the growing concern that people with learning disabilities and autistic people experience poorer health and die prematurely. Whilst there has been an increase in life expectancy for people with learning disabilities over the last few years, overall this has been slow and health inequities remain. Addressing issues of intersectionality must be understood and tackled to reduce the 'double discrimination' individuals experience. The LeDeR policy and programme offers a standardised approach to carrying out reviews and aims to provide a summary of actions that need to take place to improve care. Policy change can assist in making strategic changes, but the role of individual practitioners is vital in affecting change for individuals and their families. The information gathered from LeDeR reviews relates to individuals who were loved; they were brothers, sons, nieces, daughters, grandchildren and sisters and it is in their memory that all services and individuals working across the health, social and education system have an obligation to improve services to reduce avoidable deaths and premature mortality.

References

Emerson, E. & Baines, S. (2011) Health inequalities and people with learning disabilities in the UK. *Tizard Learning Disability Review*, *16*(1), 42–48. Available at: https://doi.org/10.5042/tldr.2011.0008 (Accessed 20.5.24)

Hassiotis, A. (2020) The intersectionality of ethnicity/race and intellectual and developmental disabilities: impact on health profiles, service access and mortality. *Journal of Mental Health Research in Intellectual Disabilities*, *13*(3), 171–173. Available at: https://doi.org/10.1080/19315864.2020.1790702 (Accessed 19.5.24)

Heslop, P., Blair, Peter S., Fleming, P., Hoghton, M., Marriott, A. & Russ, L. (2014) The confidential inquiry into premature deaths of people with intellectual disabilities in the UK: a population-based study. *The Lancet*, *383*(9920), 889–895. Available at: https://doi.org/10.1016/S0140-6736(13)62026-7 (Accessed 19.5.24)

Heslop, P., Byrne, V., Calkin, R., Gielnik, K. & Huxor, A. (2022) Establishing a national mortality review programme for people with intellectual disabilities: The experience in England. *Journal of Intellectual Disabilities*, *26*(1), 264–280. Available at: https://doi.org/10.1177/1744629520970365 (Accessed 19.5.24)

Martin, K. R., Zhou, W., Bowman, M. J., Shih, J., Au, K. S., Dittenhafer-Reed, K. E., Sisson, K. A., Koeman, J., Weisenberger, D. J., Cottingham, S. L., Deroos, S. T., Devinsky, O., Winn, M. E., Cherniack, A. D., Shen, H., Northrup, H., Krueger, D. A. & Mackeigan, J. P. (2017) The genomic landscape of tuberous sclerosis complex. *Nature Communications*, *8*(1), 15816–15816. https://doi.org/10.1038/ncomms15816 (Accessed 19.5.24)

Mason, D., Ingham, B., Urbanowicz, A., Michael, C., Birtles, H., Woodbury-Smith, M., Brown, T., James, I., Scarlett, C., Nicolaidis, C. & Parr, J. R. (2019) A systematic review of what barriers and facilitators prevent and enable physical healthcare services access for autistic adults. *Journal of Autism and Developmental Disorders*, *49*(8), 338–3400. Available at: https://doi.org/10.1177/1362361321993709 (Accessed 19.5.24)

NHS Digital (2023) *Health and Care of People with Learning Disabilities: Experimental Statistics 2017–18 to 2021–22*. Available at: https://app.powerbi.com/view?r=eyJrIjoiNTYyNDM4MGYtZDRmYi00NTAxLTkzY2QtMjcwZTY2YTQ0MzNkIiwidCI6IjUwZjYwNzFmLWJiZmUtNDAxYS04ODAzLTY3Mzc0OGU2MjllMiIsImMiOjh9 (Accessed 15.5.24)

NHSE (2021) *Learning from Lives And Deaths – People with a Learning Disability and Autistic People (LeDer) Policy 2021*. https://www.england.nhs.uk/wp-content/uploads/2021/03/B0428-LeDeR-policy-2021.pdf (Accessed 12.5.2024)

NHS England (n.d.) *Who Is Involved in LeDeR*. https://www.england.nhs.uk/learning-disabilities/improving-health/learning-from-lives-and-deaths/who-is-involved/ (Accessed 12.5.2024)

O'Nions, E., Lewer, D., Petersen, I., Brown, J., Buckman, J. E. J., Charlton, R., Cooper, C., El Baou, C., Happé, F., Manthorpe, J., McKechnie, D. G. J., Richards, M., Saunders, R., Zanker, C., Mandy, W. & Stott, J. (2024) Estimating life expectancy and years of life lost for autistic people in the UK: a matched cohort study. *The Lancet Regional Health. Europe*, 36, 1–13. Available at: https://doi.org/10.1016/j.lanepe.2023.100776 (Accessed 19.5.24)

O'Nions, E., Petersen, I., Buckman, J. E. J., Charlton, R., Cooper, C., Corbett, A., Happé, F., Manthorpe, J., Richards, M., Saunders, R., Zanker, C., Mandy, W. & Stott, J. (2023). Autism in England: assessing underdiagnosis in a population-based cohort study of prospectively collected primary care data. *The Lancet Regional Health. Europe*, 29, 1–13. Available at: https://doi.org/10.1016/j.lanepe.2023.100626 (Accessed 20.5.24)

Public Health England (2023) *Learning Disability – Applying All Our Health*. https://www.gov.uk/government/publications/learning-disability-applying-all-our-health/learning-disabilities-applying-all-our-health (Accessed 12.5.2024)

Robertson, J., Raghavan, R., Emerson, E., Baines, S. & Hatton, C. (2019) What do we know about the health and health care of people with intellectual disabilities from minority ethnic groups in the United Kingdom? A systematic review. *Journal of Applied Research Intellectual Disabilities*, 32, 1310–1334. Available at: https://doi.org/10.1111/jar.12630 (Accessed 19.5.24)

Rubin, I. L., Merrick, J., Greydanus, D. E. & Patel, D. R. (eds) (2016) *Health Care for People with Intellectual and Developmental Disabilities Across the Lifespan*. Cham: Springer International Publishing AG.

Salmi, D. (2023) People with learning disabilities can face double discrimination: people from black, Asian and minority ethnic backgrounds who also have learning disabilities face higher levels of healthcare inequalities. *Learning Disability Practice*, 26(3), 12–14. Available at: https://doi.org/10.7748/ldp.26.3.12.s4 (Accessed 19.5.24)

The King's Fund (2022) *What Are Health Inequalities?* Available at: https://www.kingsfund.org.uk/publications/what-are-health-inequalities (Accessed 12.5.2024)

Umpleby, K., Roberts, C., Cooper-Moss, N., Chesterton, L., Ditzel, N., Garner, C., Clark, S., Butt, J., Hatton, C. & Chauhan, U. (2023) *We Deserve Better: Ethnic Minorities with a Learning Disability and Barriers to Healthcare*. Race and Health Observatory Report. Available at: https://www.nhsrho.org/wp-content/uploads/2023/05/Part-A-RHO-LD-Policy-Data-Review-Report.pdf (Accessed 19.5.24)

White, A., Sheehan, R., Ding, J., Roberts, C., Magill, N., Keagan-Bull, R., Carter, B., Ruane, M., Xiang, X., Chauhan, U., Tuffrey-Wijne, I. and Strydom, A. (2022) *Learning from Lives and Deaths – People with a Learning Disability and Autistic People (LeDeR) Report for 2021 (LeDeR 2021)*. Available at: https://www.kcl.ac.uk/ioppn/assets/fans-dept/leder-main-report-hyperlinked.pdf (Accessed 19.5.24)

White, A., Sheehan, R., Ding, J., Roberts, C., Magill, N., Keagan-Bull, R., Carter, B., Ruane, M., Xiang, X., Chauhan, U., Tuffrey-Wijne, I. and Strydom, A. (2023) *LeDeR Annual Report Learning from Lives and Deaths: People with a Learning Disability and Autistic People*. Available at: https://www.kcl.ac.uk/ioppn/assets/fans-dept/leder-2022-v2.0.pdf (Accessed 12.5.2024)

Williams, R., Oyinlola, J., Heslop, P. & Glover, G. (2017) Mortality rates in people with intellectual disabilities. *International Journal of Population Data Science*, 1(1). Available at: https://doi.org/10.23889/ijpds.v1i1.333 (Accessed 20.5.24)

Lived experiences and professional insights:

Understanding care and treatment for people with learning disabilities and autistic people

Inclusive communication
Creating positive outcomes – a mother's lived experience

Amanda Glennon

When I meet other parents of children who have Down's syndrome for the first time, it never takes long for the conversation to get to that question. You know the one, the question that in a sense defines our stories, the reason we had connected in the first place. The question is of course, 'How did you find out?' Simple as that. Anyone listening may think, 'Find out what?', but for us this an unspoken known. How did you find out that your son/daughter has that extra chromosome, Trisomy 21, Down's syndrome? And as we begin to share our stories – even though this has happened countless times with other parents – we are still surprised by how similar our stories are!

For me and my family, our story of receiving our daughter's diagnosis starts on 14 December 2005. However, I am going to rewind back to her birth date some five days earlier – that's important because the story I am sharing with you is not how I found out, it's about what I already knew.

So here we are on 9 December 2005. It's 9.30 a.m. and after a sleepless night my son Joe was born, followed two minutes later his twin sister, Alice. Alice was a little smaller than her twin brother who had already been placed in his dad's arms. Alice had been in distress resulting in an emergency caesarean, so I wasn't surprised that her initial checks took longer than Joe's, although it seemed forever before she was placed into my arms.

The moment I held and laid my eyes on her I thought to myself, this is Alice, relief that she suited the name we have already given her, and she has Down's syndrome. I looked around and no one said anything. In that moment I knew absolutely without doubt she had Down's syndrome, despite having no previous knowledge or experience. I was woozy and tired, but I knew I was right, though no one else seemed to notice. It was all surreal – I just waited expectantly for someone to mention something – neither in denial, nor burying my head in the sand, just waiting.

It was four days later that someone else said those two words out loud. We had ended up with a longer stay in hospital than was initially planned, and on day four paediatric consultation took us to one side and asked to do some tests. He explained

DOI: 10.4324/9781003341765-8

they would be testing for Down's syndrome. I felt relief at finally hearing someone else say those two words out loud, but he then went on to explain that he and his colleagues were sure that she didn't have 'it'. And there it was – the moment I had waited four days for – but he didn't think Alice had Down's syndrome and I knew he was wrong.

I guess this made it difficult for him the next day as he sat us down, which he did after asking the nurses to take both babies away for a while, and informed us that our daughter did indeed have Down's syndrome.

For me he was providing the professional diagnosis of something I already knew. I didn't know anything about Down's syndrome, and clearly had to get up to speed quickly to support our beautiful daughter. But here was the lesson: I should in this moment have realised my own instincts were good and I should trust them – but I didn't.

A similar thing happened many years later. From Alice being around 2 years old we suspected she was autistic, by the age of around 8 we knew for sure and at the age of 14 she finally received the formal medical diagnosis – a 12-year wait. But let's go back to Alice's early years.

In the years that followed her birth, Alice had many medical appointments, procedures and interventions. As is typical, people with Down's syndrome have the same health challenges as everyone else but there is a higher prevalence, so that meant more check-ups, more interventions and more treatments. Initially she was like any other infant sitting on her mum's knee and being held while been prodded and poked. As she became a little older it was clear her verbal communication was significantly delayed, and she relied heavily on Makaton signs and symbols to support communication.

As the twins got older, I started to notice that Alice's twin brother Joe would be talked to and included in medical appointments and – put simply – Alice was not. As soon as it was clear to the healthcare professional that Alice couldn't verbally respond, they would switch direct communication to me. They would then ask me to hold her, take her shoes off, hold her arms, hold her head in position, restrain her – and I did all this. I complied in 'doing to' Alice to complete the procedures; note: 'doing to her' *not* 'doing with her'. 'Doing to her' to get blood, to have ear moulds made, to give injections. Deep down I knew this was wrong. In the clinic and treatment rooms I stopped being Mum and became part of the medical team 'doing to' Alice.

It became a horrible cycle. If during an appointment the doctor asked for bloods, I would comply and help the team of approximately four nurses/medical staff in holding and restraining my daughter so we could take blood. Alice would get distressed, and try to remove herself from the situation, and we would hold onto her even tighter. The job usually got done, but at what cost? I would usually drive home shaking and crying, hoping that next time would just be better, but it wasn't – until one day the cycle was broken.

The cycle was broken by Alice herself, getting bigger and stronger, and having the will to no longer consent to being 'done to'. She simply downed tools and refused – she refused to go into the treatment rooms, or to be held or restrained, and the consequence was huge.

Around the time she was 10 years old Alice started having bloating and pain in her stomach. It was quickly diagnosed as coeliac disease. Coeliac disease had similar symptoms to H-Pylori (Helicobacter), and people with Down's syndrome are more likely to be coeliac – case closed! But to register as coeliac we needed a blood test, and we couldn't get one, because Alice refused. After years of having blood tests done to her, she decided enough was enough. It was a long drawn-out 18 months going through the process of re-attempting blood tests, even attempting (unsuccessfully) to sedate her and take bloods. Deep down I wanted to insist we went straight to an exploratory investigation under general anaesthetic, but the healthcare professionals were the experts, and I was complicit in following the protocol – no reasonable adjustments were suggested and I didn't ask for any.

When Alice finally had that exploratory investigation it was discovered that she was not coeliac but had H. pylori. In fact she had several nasty gastric ulcers causing discomfort and bloating – and she had had this for 18 months. It hit me like a ton of bricks.

Years of negative outcomes and being 'done to' absolutely leads to more serious health implications in the longer term. Our adult population with learning disabilities, autism and/or communication difficulties are exposed to this higher risk, and it is not acceptable.

I hadn't learnt from my earlier lesson to trust my instincts. My instincts were telling me I should not comply with these interventions that were resulting in repeated negative experiences for Alice. It was time for change.

At this time, I was involved in the development of a book called *Going to Hospital*. *Going to Hospital* is a book that helps prepare children for their visit to hospital. A simple picture book with some functional signs and symbols to support understanding. It became my vehicle for change. The book and resources gave me a way to start the dialogue with Alice's healthcare teams.

When Alice was scheduled for surgery I contacted the hospital with a draft copy of the book and asked some questions: Did they have a learning disability nurse available? Was there anyone who could support Alice through her visit with Makaton signs and symbols? Who would be there to communicate with her when she woke up scared and alone in recovery? It worked – the hospital printed out the resources and made sure a member of the team was able to sign to Alice and support her procedure with a visual symbol timeline. Alice was nil by mouth, but what does that mean to a person with a learning disability/autism that has never heard the phrase? Alice was given a schedule, which rather than telling her she couldn't eat or drink showed instead when she could; this was key in supporting Alice's understanding. This permanent visual supported her independence, anxiety and need for knowledge of now and next. The procedure was a huge success, so much so that an image of Alice getting ready for surgery with a symbol timeline was included in the final version of the book.

Buoyed by this positive outcome Alice and I started turning up for appointments armed with copies of the book and the Makaton resources. We gave them out to paediatricians, GPs, nurses, play therapists, dentists. The biggest impact they had was that the communication moved directly to Alice. When the paediatrician asked for an unplanned blood test, we would look in the book with Alice and discuss it. Alice would decide if she was happy to have a test that day or choose to come back another time – Alice's choice.

I felt less pressured to comply with the timings of the medical team and go with Alice's decision. I started to make sure staff would ask her consent to every step of the process, simply offering a Makaton sign for yes or no. If Alice said no, we would need to honour that and stop – arranging to come back another day to try again. There were very few occasions we needed to do that though as Alice would usually say yes; just being asked and feeling in control made a huge difference resulting in positive outcomes.

Don't get me wrong: having the patient agree doesn't always mean the procedure will be straightforward. Take blood tests for example. Alice would now give consent to a blood test but often the nurse could not find blood as Alice's veins are deep. This confused and worried Alice in equal measure – why didn't she have blood, was something wrong? The reasonable adjustment for this was to take the sample from the back of Alice's hand – the nurses were worried about this. How can we hold down her hand while we do this, they asked. My reply was that you don't need to restrain or hold her hand down, you just need to ask her if you can do it – if she says yes, she will let you do it.

They were not very confident I could see, but Alice made me proud as she does every day, by agreeing and resting her hand and holding still while the blood sample was taken, another positive outcome. I am so proud of Alice, and that she has been able to overcome the impacts of those early negative outcomes. We are in a place now where I know if we needed a blood sample, Alice would allow it.

It has been a long journey – hopefully one that others will not need to take, that's down to you ensuring direct communication and inclusive environments that lead to positive outcomes from the very start.

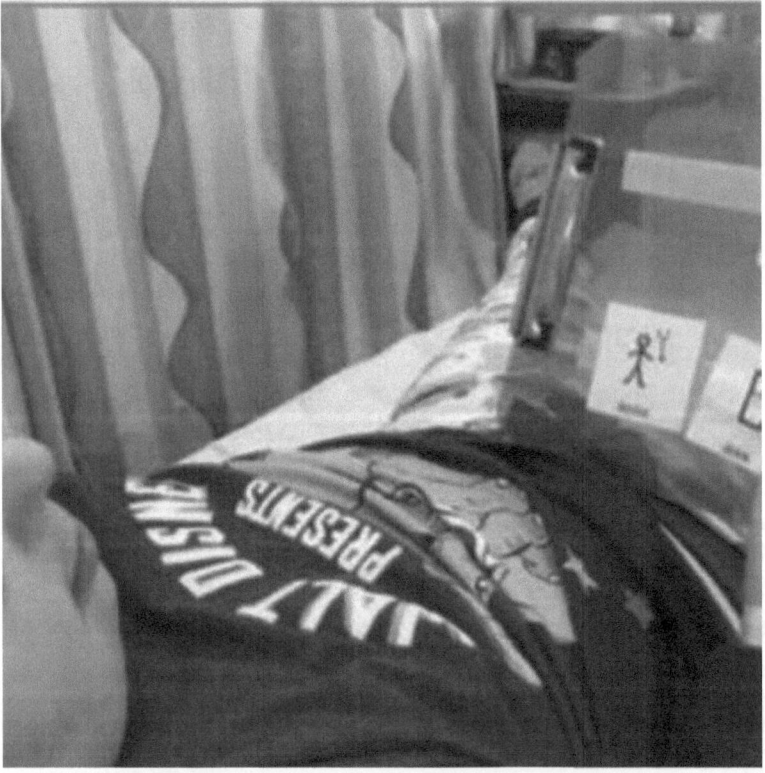

FIGURE 6.1 Alice using Makaton

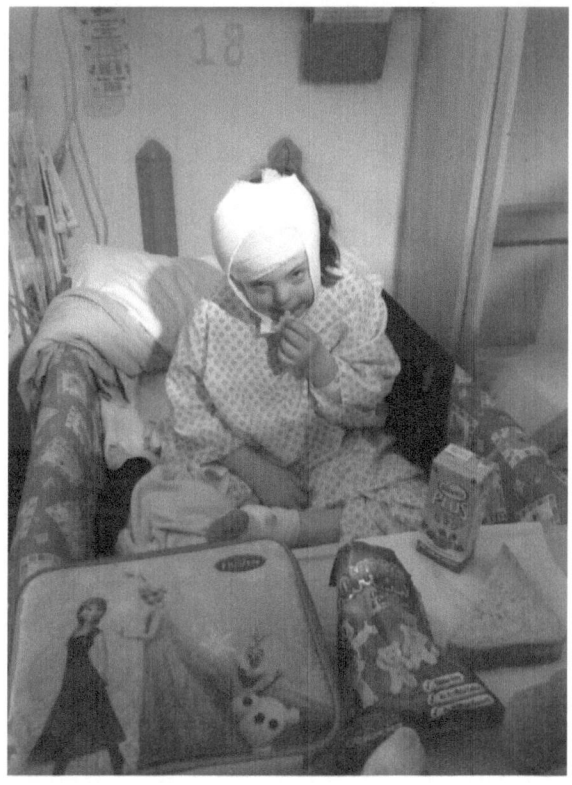

FIGURE 6.2 Alice in nursing bay

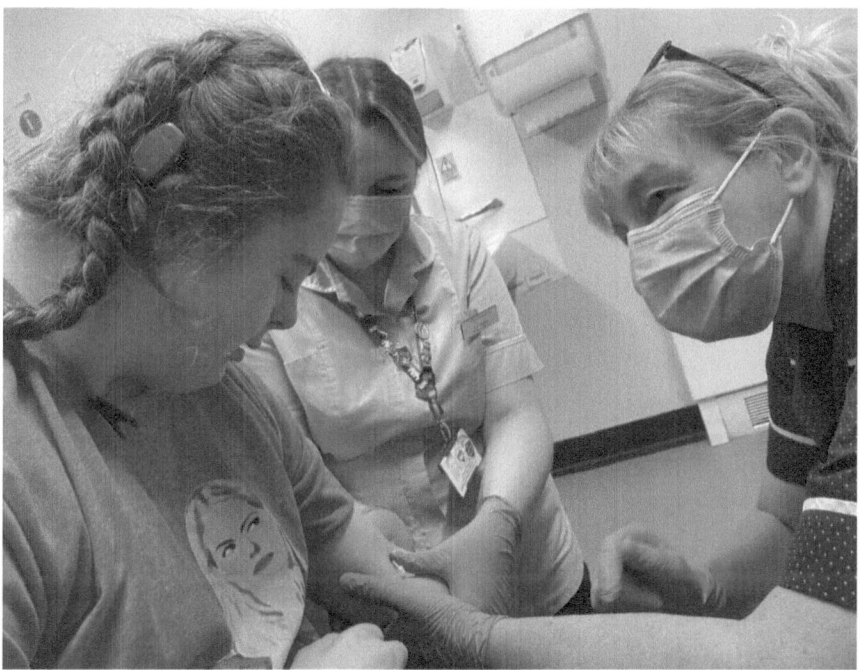

FIGURE 6.3 Alice having an injection

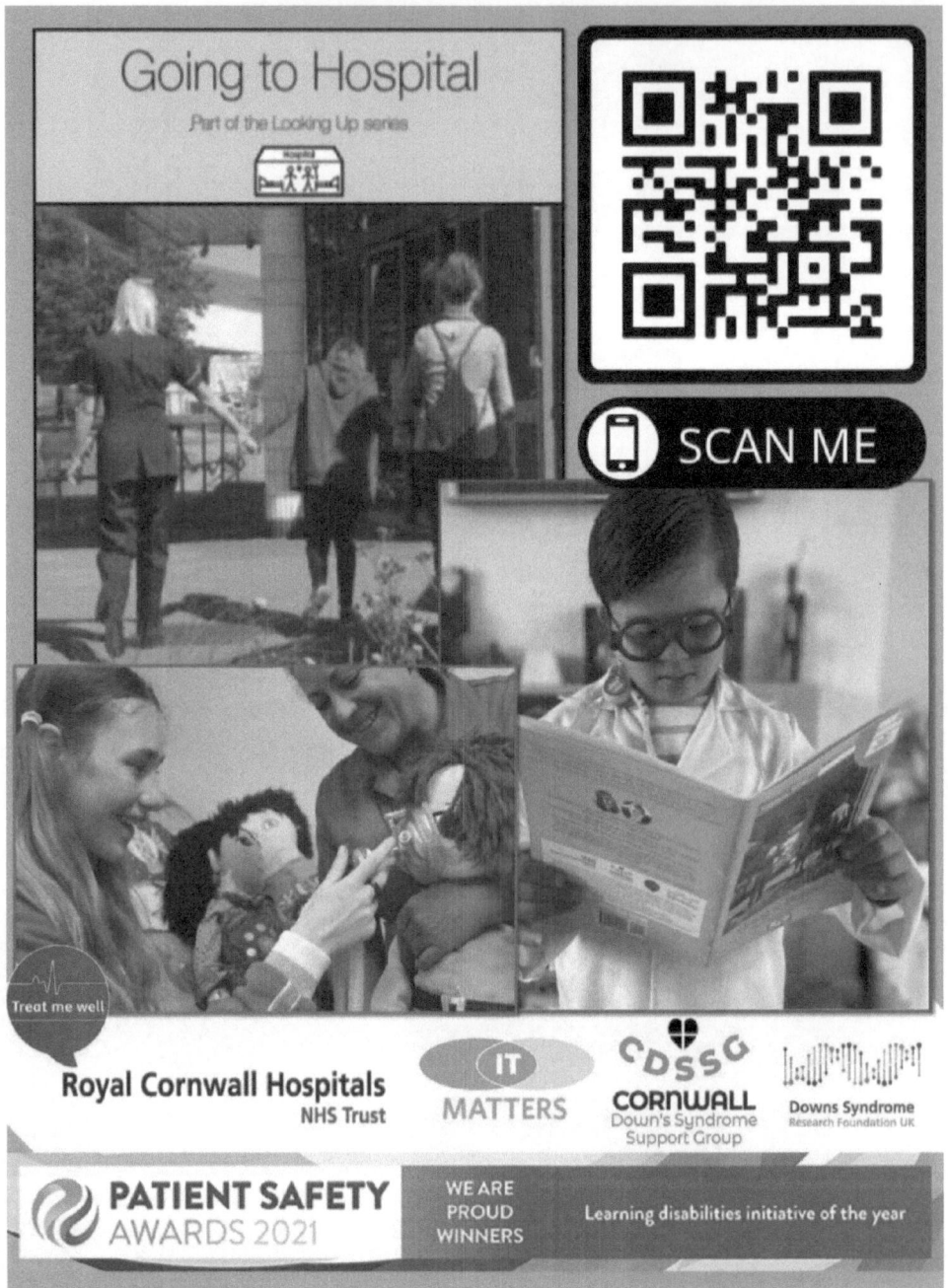

FIGURE 6.4 *Going to Hospital* book

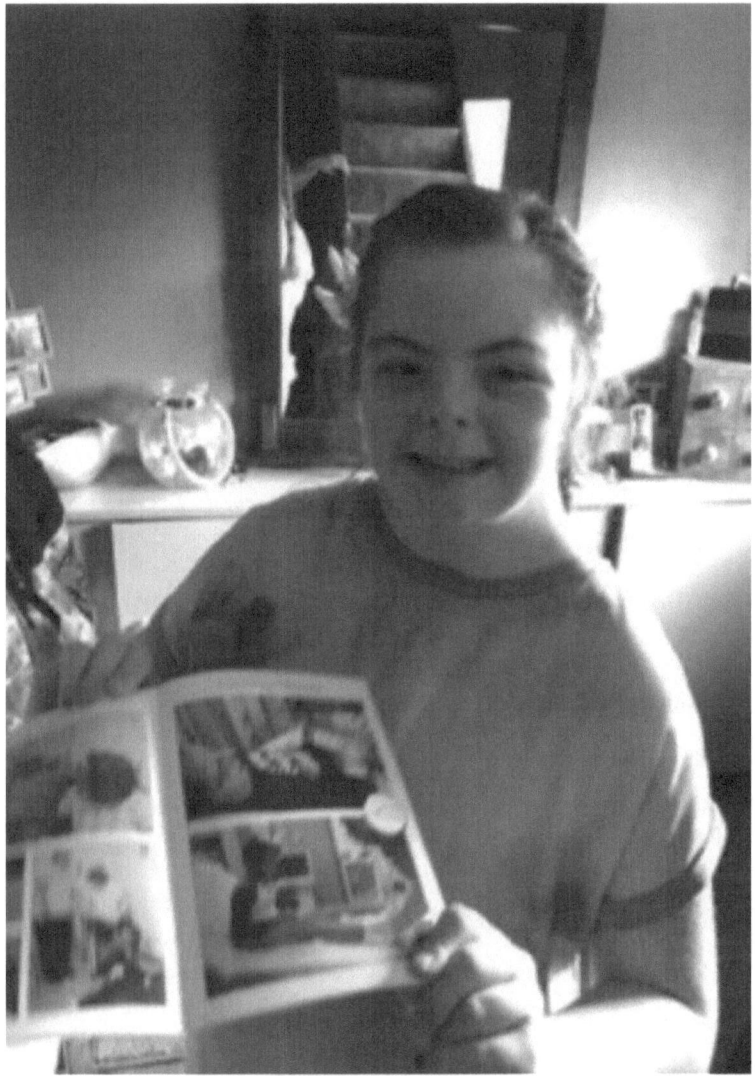

FIGURE 6.5 Alice and *Going to Hospital* book

Further resources

There are many good resources freely available to support you. Take a look at www. Makaton.org. There is a library with free healthcare resources focusing on direct and inclusive patient communication.

Cornwall Down's Syndrome Support Group (CDSSG) *Going to Hospital* book. Available at: https://www.cdssg.org.uk/going-to-hospital-book/

NHS Accessible Information Standard (n.d.) Available at: https://www.england. nhs.uk/about/equality/equality-hub/patient-equalities-programme/equality-frameworks-and-information-standards/accessibleinfo/

7

Autism and learning disabilities

Linda Woodcock

According to NHS England a significant number of autistic people also have a learning disability. People with a learning disability and autistic people will experience the same illnesses, traumas, accidents and so on as the general population but research shows that people with a learning disability have higher rates of death from avoidable causes than for the general population, (49% vs 22%) and die at a younger age (LeDeR Report 2021). There is also evidence that premature mortality is even higher for autistic people compared to the general population (at least 12 years) (Hirvikoski et al, 2016) and that autistic people have higher rates of health problems throughout childhood, adolescence and adulthood including a higher rate of mental health diagnoses (Lai et al, 2019). Autistic individuals may have one or more co-occurring conditions such as epilepsy, ADHD, anxiety, depression or gut issues. There are some genetic and chromosomal conditions that may have features of autism (e.g. Fragile X syndrome, Down's syndrome, Angelman syndrome, Neurofibromatosis, Cri du chat, Cornelia de Lange syndrome). This list is not exhaustive and due to diagnostic overshadowing there is often a lack of acknowledgement and understanding from clinicians that the features of autism may be present in these conditions.

What is autism?

Autism is a lifelong neurodevelopmental difference. It is a neurodivergent condition which means the brain works differently from non-autistic (often referred to as neurotypical) people. This influences the way a person experiences their senses, how they communicate and interact with others, and how they think and process information. Autistic people are more likely to feel stressed and anxious due to their different sensory experiences, communication differences and confusion around understanding other people and societal expectations. They may have difficulty in recognising and understanding their own emotions and expressing their emotions; this is known as alexithymia (present in 40–65% of autistic individuals).

We all suffer stress to different degrees and levels of severity and we all get anxious sometimes. However, neurotypical people generally realise when they are becoming

DOI: 10.4324/9781003341765-9

stressed or anxious and can take positive steps to relieve this, using coping strategies developed over their lifetime. Whereas neurotypical people may wake up each morning with quite low levels of anxiety, an autistic person may start their day with a much higher level of stress and anxiety. They may not have developed coping strategies, and this means that they may reach crisis point more quickly than others.

Autistic individuals rely on and thrive on **structure**, and they find safety in **predictability** in what is often seems a chaotic and unpredictable world. To combats these feelings of anxiety and stress, offering structure which is meaningful to the individual is paramount as this will help give predictability to their day and interactions. Visual support such as timetables, pictures and symbols tailored to the individual's preferences and developmental ability should be readily available.

Autistic individuals may also use a variety of methods to self-soothe (known as stimming), this could manifest itself as repetitive speech, movements, using familiar objects, watching or listening to familiar programmes, DVDs, music, asking repetitive questions and needing a predictable response. They may also have a focused interest which will give them pleasure and may also help them self-regulate; this may be talking about a particular subject, collecting objects, vocalising or repetitive physical movement. These stimming and self-soothing tools should not be limited as they perform a very important role in helping autistic individuals self-regulate and often give them joy.

Communication and interaction

Autistic people may communicate differently from neurotypical people. Some may be non-speaking; some may experience situational mutism (can't speak in some environments or when they're anxious or overwhelmed). The majority of autistic people with learning disabilities will struggle at times to understand spoken or written language. This means a willingness to supplement the spoken word by using objects, photographs, line drawings, symbols or sign is needed. In order to do this well, we must be person-centred. We need to know which method or combination of methods suits each person best.

Expression is the act of transferring what is inside your head – your thoughts, feelings, desires, wants and wishes – to another person. All people have individual ways of expressing themselves, and for autistic people with learning disabilities this may mean using other methods than speech alone. Again objects, photographs, line drawings, symbols, signing and/or body language may be used to express information. All of these are equally valid forms of expression and need to be interpreted as such.

Often neurotypical people struggle to connect with autistic individuals and vice versa. This lack of understanding of each other has led to educationalists and clinicians devising behavioural plans to try and modify what they see as a lack of social skills; the message that autistic people receive is that they are not good enough and have to be more like their neurotypical counterparts. Instead of trying to 'fix' autistic people, we should put our efforts into understanding their experiences and offering support which shows an acceptance for who they are and a respect for their ways of socialising and communicating.

TOP TIPS

Communication

- Simplify your language
- Give one instruction at a time, not a sequence
- Keep facial expressions and gestures simple and clear
- Give the person time to respond
- Use additional visual support to help a person understand and make their needs known
- Be sensitive to the person's attempt to communicate
- Say what you mean and mean what you say
- Use concrete language and avoid metaphors
- Allow for processing time
- Set up situations which will encourage the person to attempt to communicate

Social interaction

- Understand that the person may feel threatened by the close proximity of others
- Allow for solitariness
- Go at the person's pace when trying to develop interaction
- Identify what the person likes and dislikes socially – use this knowledge when planning activities
- The person is more likely to interact with familiar people, so give them time to get to know you and don't confuse them with changes in personnel
- It takes time to build positive relationships

Low-arousal approaches

- Offer maximum consistency of approach
- Help the person develop predictable routines to reduce anxiety
- Introduce any changes gradually
- Carry out an environmental audit and make changes to help reduce sensory distress
- Help explain changes by giving visual clues
- Don't break promises
- Be aware of your own arousal levels and remain calm
- If the person becomes agitated, understand that the usual strategies for calming may have the opposite effect and distress them even more
- If the person has a focused interest, do not try to stop it – see it as positive and make sure they have access to it.

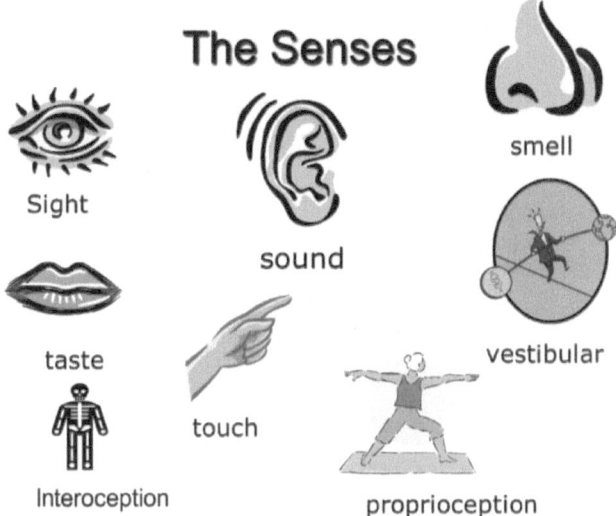

FIGURE 7.1 The senses

Sensory perception – involves the systems of sensing through which information about the world and ourselves is gathered, i.e. sight, hearing, touch, taste and smell. **Processing** – relates to the way in which information is decoded and how it is interpreted by the brain. Autistic individuals have a different sensory experience from non-autistic people. Although each autistic person's experience is unique to them, they are likely to have heightened sensory awareness in some areas and may require more sensory stimulus in other areas. If they are hypersensitive they might find the sensory input overwhelming and even painful and if they are hyposensitive they may seek out sensory stimulus.

Clinical settings can be very challenging for anyone experiencing sensory hypersensitivity. There are countless examples of autistic people being very ill with painful or life-threatening illnesses or dislocated or broken limbs which have been missed or dismissed by health professional due to the differing sensory experience and expression of pain combined with communication issues.

Dr Emma Goodall, an autistic author and research fellow, has written about interoception which is an internal sensory system that informs us when we are hungry and when we want to go to the toilet, but also when we are becoming angry or upset. She argues that the development of interoception can slow down or even stop in autistic people although it is not known why. She says:

> As an example, when I am overwhelmed I am much more easily distressed by small sensory things. I often have no idea what emotions I am experiencing. When in this state, I am less able to self-manage my eating or drinking as I do not notice nor recognise my body signals of hunger and thirst. I am also less able to self-regulate my emotions as I am not aware of the emotion that is developing and so cannot respond helpfully. This means anxiety may skyrocket before I realise I am anxious. At this point I have no idea what will help

manage my anxiety, whereas normally I would do some interoception activities, such as belly breathing or toe curls, to self-calm and decrease my anxiety.

('Interoception and mental wellbeing in autistic people', https://www.autism.org.uk/advice-and-guidance/professional-practice/interoception-wellbeing, March 2022)

Common sensory distress in a clinical setting

- Noisy waiting rooms
- Lack of safe quiet spaces
- A dislike of people getting too close
- A fear of being in an enclosed space, combined with loud operational noise of scanners, etc.
- Finding physical touch unpleasant or distressing
- The smell or feel of rubber gloves
- The smell of disinfectants, antiseptics, etc.
- The feel of hospital gowns
- Tight things such as blood pressure cuffs
- Some medical equipment will be hard and cold
- A dislike of bright lights, especially if they are shining in eyes
- A fear or dislike having blood taken
- Difficulty swallowing tablets
- Difficulty with the smell and taste of certain medications

When working with autistic individuals we need to understand the impact their sensory differences have on their health and wellbeing. Sensory and emotional overload, too many demands and frustration due to not having the necessary means of communication can leave the individual so distressed that they may enter a state of either meltdown or shutdown. Having a plan taking all things into account is vital.

The use of **hospital passports**, a document prepared in collaboration with the individual and those that know them best is the most effective way of ensuring that everyone involved in their care is aware of their personal needs. Their medical history, communication preferences, sensory profile, likely triggers for anxiety, and likes and dislikes should all be documented.

The passport should also include a 'Ways to help me avoid distress' section, for example:

- Can you cope with bright lights if you are given warning and support – what sort of support?

- Can you cope with the unpleasant noise(s) if you are given warning and support – what sort of support?

- Can you cope with tight things if you are given warning and support – what sort of support?

- Can you cope with having your blood taken if you are given warning and support – what sort of support? Does anaesthetic cream help?

- Can you cope with enclosed spaces if you are given warning and support – what sort of support? Would 'calming' medication help?

Many NHS Trusts have templates which can be used by staff. NHS England has one in a downloadable format: https://www.england.nhs.uk/publication/health-and-care-passports/

Mental health settings

For autistic adults with a learning disability the experience of being an inpatient is likely to be one of confusion and fear, and the misunderstanding of their responses to stressful situations may lead to overmedication, physical restraint and isolation. The impact of these interventions is one of continuing trauma. Many will go on to experience post-traumatic stress disorder (PTSD). An inpatient ward is likely to be a very stressful environment with other patients who may also be distressed, staff members who may have little knowledge of the individual, unpredictable changes, lack of safe space for the individual to withdraw to, lack of appropriate communication tools, structure and consistency of staff. There may be rigid blanket bans on items deemed unsafe but which may be essential to the individual to help them self-soothe and regulate.

Meltdown and shutdowns

When an autistic individual experiences sensory, emotional or social overwhelm they may experience meltdown or shutdown; they are two sides of the same coin – it is when the stress and anxiety of a situation exceeds their ability to cope. *It is important to note that they are both outside of the individual's control.* Meltdown will put the individual into flight or flight mode and if they are not given the opportunity to escape to a safe place to calm down and self-regulate, the meltdown could escalate into shouting, aggression to others, self-injury or damage to their environment. This behaviour is often misinterpreted and may result in restrictive practices such as over-medication, isolation or restraint. We should not locate the problem purely with the individual, but see it in the context of a response to environmental factors and not having their needs met, which are causing the distress.

When a shutdown occurs the individual may become withdrawn, lose ability to self-care, stop speaking or responding to others. They may not be able to remove themselves from the stressful situation.

The over-medication of autistic individuals is well documented. This has led to the establishment of the STOMP/STAMP initiative:

■   STOMP = STopping the Over-Medication of People with a learning disability, autism or both

■   STAMP = Supporting Treatment and Appropriate Medication in Paediatrics

STOMP was introduced in 2016 to reduce the use of psychotropic medication in both community and hospital settings. STOMP-STAMP was launched in 2018, for children and young people with learning disability and/or autism diagnosis.

Most psychotropic medication administered to people with learning disability and/or autism diagnosis is given for behaviours of concern – to children as well as adults.

All healthcare providers who prescribe psychotropic medicine to children and young people with a learning disability, autism or both are asked to adopt the STAMP healthcare pledge. The goal is to improve the quality of life of people with a learning disability, autism or both by reducing the potential harm of inappropriate psychotropic drugs.

This includes where medication is being used wholly inappropriately, as a 'chemical restraint' to control behaviours of concern.

Working with families

We have to acknowledge that there is often conflict and tension between families and professionals. Understanding the family journey is crucial and development of positive relationships is essential and takes work.

Staff in stretched services have less time to get to know the individual admitted to the ward. Therefore, the in-depth and long-term knowledge that carers have is invaluable in helping others to understand their loved one and yet often this resource is underused. There is a need for better consultation between staff and carers. Establishing a good relationship has to be worked on, but this relational aspect is hampered by a number of things, such as people enacting power imbalances between carers and staff (e.g. use of professional terminology that sets up an 'experts and the rest' divide and exclude people, a paternalistic culture and carers feeling they needed permission to be involved).

Confidentiality is often cited as a barrier. Carers recognise the right to confidentiality that it is a difficult area, Some, though, feel that the issue has been misused to exclude carers, more through misinterpretation than deliberate exclusion. This is particularly difficult for those carers of patients who have an additional learning disability. They may have spent a lifetime caring and advocating for, and protecting and representing their loved one and they are often left bewildered and frustrated when faced with the usually unplanned admission and find themselves excluded from all aspects of their care.

For many the feeling of guilt and loss they experience can be devastating. They may feel that that they have failed their loved one and they are no longer able to protect them from what is often a hostile environment. The feeling of devastation only grows as visiting their loved one in a secure environment and seeing their distress stays with them until the next quite often unsatisfactory visit. We must remember that for all the time before the admission often the only constant in the individual's life was family and on discharge this will also be true. If the experience is a negative one which sadly is often the case, the trauma for both family and the individual will stay with them. Building positive and trusting relationships between staff and families takes time and effort, The hope is that with understanding, empathy and commitment, the outcome can be very different.

NHS England have produced a clinical guide for frontline staff to support the management of patients with a learning disability and autism. Below are the main points, which should be addressed when assessing and treating a patient with a learning disability or autistic person:

- **Be aware of diagnostic overshadowing:** This occurs when the symptoms arising from physical or mental ill health are misattributed to a person's learning disability or autism leading to delayed diagnosis or treatment. People with a learning disability and autistic people have the same illnesses as everyone else, but the way that they respond to or communicate their symptoms may be different and not obvious.

- **Pay attention to healthcare passports:** Some people with a learning disability and some autistic people have a healthcare passport giving information about the person and their health needs, preferred method of communication and other preferences. Ask the person or their accompanying carer if they have one of these.

- **Ensure that clinical decisions around care and access to treatment are made on an individual basis:** People should not have a DNACPR (do not attempt cardiopulmonary resuscitation) recorded on their clinical record simply because they have a learning disability or are autistic. Every person has individual needs and preferences which must be taken account of, and they should always have high-quality standards of care. It is also important not to make generalised judgements or assumptions about people's vulnerability or frailty based on their dependence on others for support in daily living.

- **Listen to parents and carers:** Families and carers have a wealth of information about the individual and how their health has been, including any comorbidities and the medication that the person is taking. Listen to them as well as the person you are caring for. They know the person well and how to look after them when they are not in hospital. They also know how the person's current behaviour may differ from usual, as an indication that they are unwell. The family or carer may have short videos of the person to give you an idea of their usual self. Remember that the carer they come into hospital with may not be their usual carer at this unusual time. You may wish to talk to their usual carer as soon as is practicable.

- **Make reasonable adjustments:** It is a legal requirement to make reasonable adjustments to care for people with a disability under the Equality Act (2010).

Getting the reasonable adjustments right is important to help you make the correct diagnostic and treatment decisions for an individual. You can ask the person and their carer or family member what reasonable adjustments should be made. Adjustments aim to remove barriers, do things in a different way, or to provide something additional to enable a person to receive the assessment and treatment they need. Possible examples include allocating a clinician by gender, taking blood samples by thumb prick rather than needle, providing a quiet space to see the patient away from excess noise and activity.

- **Communication:** Communicate with and try to understand the person you are caring for. Check with the person themselves, their family member or carer or in their hospital or communication passport for the best way to achieve this. Use simple, clear language, avoiding medical terms and 'jargon' wherever possible. Some people may be non-verbal and unable to tell you how they feel. Pictures may be a useful way of communicating with some people, but not all.

- **Understanding behavioural responses to illness, pain and discomfort:** A person with a learning disability and some autistic people may not be able to articulate their response to pain in the expected way: for example, they may say that they have a pain in their stomach when the pain is not there; may say the pain is less acute than you would anticipate; or not say they are in pain when they are. Some may feel pain in a different way or respond to it differently: for example, by displaying challenging behaviour; laughing or crying; trying to hurt themselves; or equally may become withdrawn or quiet. People who use a wheelchair may have chronic pain. Understanding what is 'normal' for that person by talking to them, their family and carers is crucial to helping with assessment and diagnosis. You can use pictures to help establish whether a person is in pain and where that pain is.

- **Mental Capacity Act (2005):** People with a learning disability and autistic people should be assumed to have capacity in line with the principles of the Mental Capacity Act. Assess their capacity to make a decision about their treatment or care in line with the person's communication abilities and needs and follow the principle of the Mental Capacity Act in making appropriate efforts and adjustment to enable decision making wherever possible. Remember that capacity is time and decision-specific. Refer to the MCA Code of Practice for guidance.

- **Ask for specialist support and advice if necessary:** Your hospital learning disability team or liaison nurse can help you with issues of communication, reasonable adjustments and assessment of pain. You may also want to make contact with your local community learning disability team if your Trust does not have a learning disability liaison nurse.

- **Training on how to support people with a learning disability and autistic people:** The Oliver McGowan Mandatory Training on Learning Disability and Autism is the government's preferred and recommended training for health and social care staff. Access the e-learning on: https://www.e-lfh.org.uk/programmes/the-oliver-mcgowan-mandatory-training-on-learning-disability-and-autism/.

■ **Mental wellbeing and emotional distress:** It is estimated that 40% of people with a learning disability experience mental health problems (https://www.nice.org.uk/guidance/ng54) and research suggests autistic people may be more likely to experience depression than non-autistic people (https://www.autism.org.uk/advice-and-guidance/topics/mental-health/depression). Change in routine can have a big effect on people's emotional and mental wellbeing. A hospital setting may make people with a learning disability and autistic people more anxious or lead to adverse behaviours, such as hurting other people, hurting themselves or damaging property. Do not assume that this is an indication of mental illness and do your best to work with the person who is unwell, their carer or family member to find out how best to keep them calm and relaxed.

Useful links

https://www.autism.org.uk/advice-and-guidance/topics/physical-health/my-health-passport

https://www.autism.org.uk/advice-and-guidance/topics/physical-health/my-health-passport

NHS England » Clinical guide for front line staff to support the management of patients with a learning disability and autistic people – relevant to all clinical specialties

https://www.twinkl.nl/teaching-wiki/spell-autism-framework

https://www.england.nhs.uk/publication/health-and-care-passports/

8

Nursing observations and people with a learning disability
Considerations

*Helen Clarke, Melanie Wakeman, Andrea Page
and Samantha Salmon*

What are nursing observations?

Nursing students and apprentices are taught a range of core nursing skills during their nurse training course. These include nursing observations such as taking manual blood pressure, tympanic temperature and pulse, and assessing an individual's respiration. Some nursing text books refer to these skills as clinical measurement and others refer to them as clinical procedures, such as Delves-Yates (2022) and within the Royal Marsden manual of clinical nursing procedures (Lister, Hofland and Grafton, 2020). Students and apprentices are also supported in carrying out these skills while on placement by their practice assessors and practice supervisors.

These observations enable nursing students and apprentices to detect changes in the individual's condition quickly and accurately. They can be reported to practice assessors and supervisors on placement so that appropriate actions can be decided. Undertaking nursing observations is a fundamental element of care.

Nursing observations should not be taken in isolation; nurses, doctors, nursing students and apprentices need to know the appropriate clinical ranges for their patient population, and also child or adult ranges. However, determining whether findings are 'normal' for the age of the individual may be problematic with some patients who have a learning disability.

What is the issue?

The seminal book *Physical Health of Adults with Intellectual Disabilities* (Prasher and Janicki, 2002) has established that 'much of our knowledge regarding physical health issues in adults with a learning disability is based primarily on generalisations from clinical and research findings on the general population'. There is a lack of

DOI: 10.4324/9781003341765-10

research on whether profound or multiple learning disabilities affects observation findings for some individuals (Page and Wakeman, 2017). Folch et al. (2017) and Northway and Hopes (2022) identify that certain physical health conditions are more prevalent among people with a learning disability, such as urinary incontinence, oral problems, chronic bronchitis, thyroid problems, heart disease, liver disease and strokes. The Care Quality Commission (CQC) was referred to in mainstream media (BBC, 2020) and revealed that there had been a 134% increase in deaths in people with a learning disability in England during the coronavirus pandemic, stating: 'We already know that people with a learning disability are at an increased risk of respiratory illnesses, meaning that access to testing could be key to reducing infection and saving lives' (Kate Terroni, CQC).

Most textbooks mention factors that affect readings, such as posture, exercise and neural mechanisms. We have found none that consider the potential physiological impact of having a learning disability, and in particular the impact that a profound and multiple learning disability may have on the individual. This means that the age-related ranges for each nursing observation may not be correct for your patient who has a learning disability For example, the 'normal' adult range for counting respiration is 12–18 breaths per minute. But this may not be correct for your patient who has a learning disability.

What does this mean for a person with a learning disability?

This means there is often no baseline data taken when the individual is well, and it is questionable to place so much emphasis on the readings being 'inside or outside' the normal clinical ranges, as such ranges may be inaccurate for the individual. This could mean the whole process of taking, recording and acting on a nursing observation may be flawed for some individuals. To prevent this, the technical data from nursing observations needs to be combined with other data, in this case consideration of the variations that altered physiology may have for the individual and how it affects the nursing observation taken.

Your considerations will include questioning whether the parameters for an individual the same age as your patient who has a learning disability apply and which technique will be most appropriate to obtain the nursing observation measurement.

The figures below highlight possible altered physiological considerations for nursing observations routinely undertaken (**respiration, pulse, temperature and blood pressure**). We have chosen to follow the ABC approach to highlight the considerations as this is the approach used with resuscitation that many of you will have been taught or through using a ABCDE (A–E) assessment tool to enhance the recognition of physiological abnormalities that signal deterioration (Resuscitation Council UK, 2021).

When looking at these figures, consider the potential variation for each nursing observation that you undertake:

> Would you expect the individual clinical observation parameter to be *higher*, *lower* or *within* the normal clinical range?

Remember, there are no definitive answers, hence the emphasis of the importance of taking baseline measurements when the individual is well, so that comparisons can be made when there are concerns about their physical health.

Respiration

It is important to keep the airway open and patent (in other words the individual is able to breathe). AVPU (airway, voice, pain and unresponsiveness) is a good indication of this. You may have come across ACVPU (which includes C – consciousness) and NEWs2 (Royal College of Physicians, 2017) as well.

Rationale for respiration (airway and breathing)

One example of how this can differ for people with a learning disability is in the upper airway the tongue is larger in people with Down syndrome and can lead to sleep apnoea or airway obstruction. Therefore, positioning can be vital to prevent blockages.

Respiratory diseases commonly occur in people with a learning disability and are a leading cause of death, as highlighted in several reports. Large studies such as Folch et al. (2017) have also shown an increased prevalence of asthma in people with a learning disability.

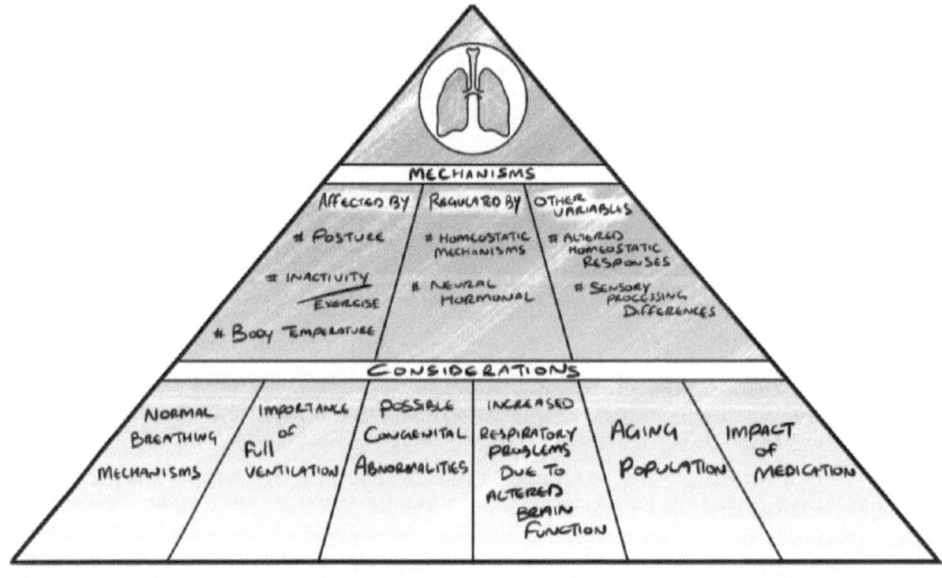

FIGURE 8.1 Respiratory image design by Matt Kelly

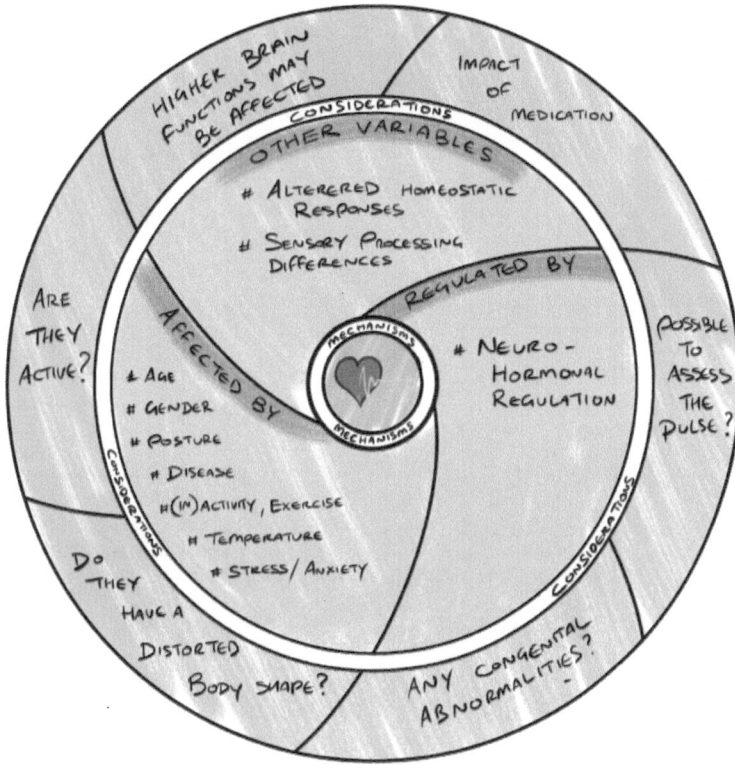

FIGURE 8.2 Pulse image design by Matt Kelly

Pulse (cardiac)

The pulse can be felt in various locations where an artery can be compressed over a bony prominence such as those in the wrist, neck and groin. The pulse rate is a quick and reliable determinant of the person's cardiovascular status, which is why pulse rates must be taken manually and not by using automated monitoring equipment.

Rationale for pulse

The pulse may be difficult to detect in the wrist and additional devices such as finger pulse oximeters may need to be used.

Blood pressure (BP) cardiac

Blood pressure is required to maintain adequate tissue and organ perfusion. It is the pressure of the circulating blood pushing against the blood vessel wall and is measured in the brachial artery in the arm using a sphygmomanometer. The systolic

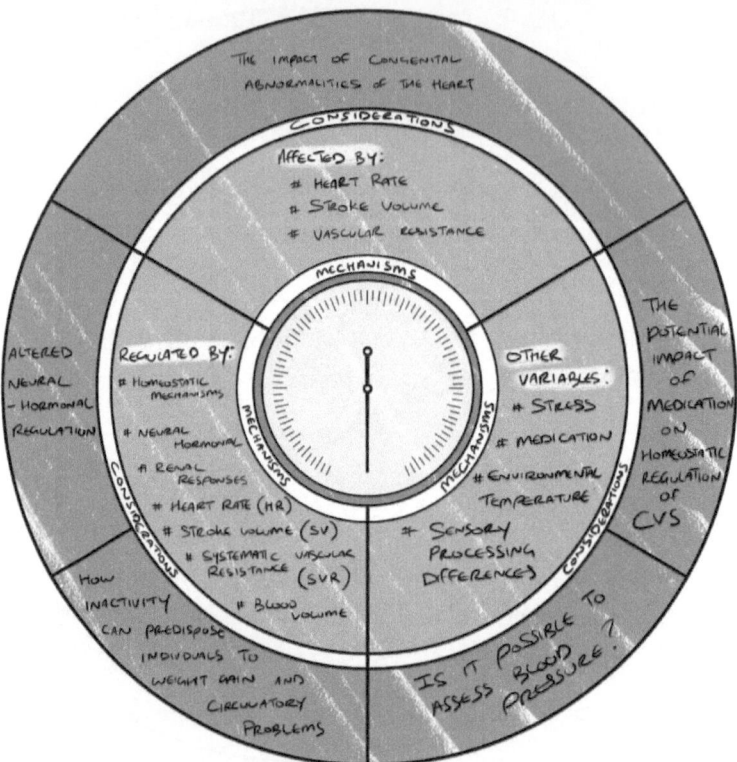

FIGURE 8.3 Blood pressure image design by Matt Kelly

pressure is when the heart contracts the diastolic pressure is when the heart is at rest. The skill of taking a blood pressure involves an inflatable cuff positioned around the individual's upper arm with a digital monitor/sphygmomanometer.

Rationale for blood pressure

Cardiac defects such as ventral septal defect (VSD) are quite common in patients who have a diagnosis of Down syndrome with one in five requiring surgery (NHS Inform 2024). The VSD would be present at birth and cause more deoxygenated blood to enter the systemic circulation. This may impact on cardiac output and blood pressure by reducing them. Cardiac drugs may be used such as inotropes to maintain blood pressure until surgery can be performed if the VSD is large and this procedure is recommended.

Temperature – disability/environment

Body temperature is a measure of how your body can make and get rid of heat.

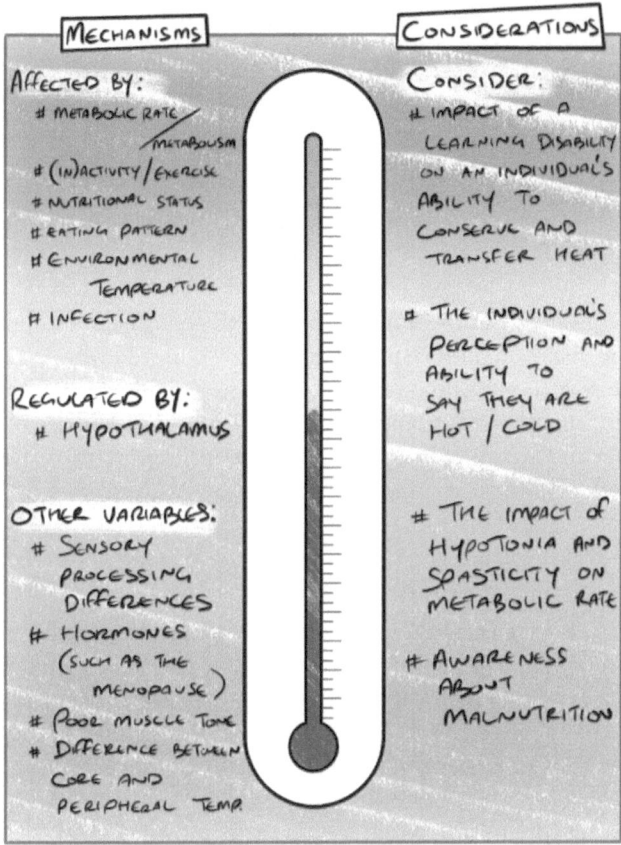

FIGURE 8.4 Temperature image design by Matt Kelly

Rationale for temperature

A high temperature may indicate the metabolic rate is faster than normal and also that the body has an increased need for energy. If the temperature is low it indicates that metabolism is slowing down.

Communication considerations

Vision and hearing issues may make communication more challenging.

For more information please go to 'Intellectual learning disability and health' website (University of Hertfordshire). This discusses specific problems and offers advice.

Also refer to article 'Eye care and people with learning disabilities: making reasonable adjustments' (Public Health England, 2020). This guide contains information about eye care and treatment for eye problems for people with learning disabilities. It also shares ideas with you about what reasonable adjustments can be made.

Appropriate communication/language to help the patient express themselves. Family integrated care can also promote better communication. Autism and sensory issues can heighten anxiety to be aware of this to minimise stimulation to allow focus, making interaction meaningful and concise as many have attention deficit disorder (ADD).

Cancers

With Down syndrome there needs to be increased cancer awareness in conditions such as leukaemia in younger groups under 4 years (Better Health, 2021). Part of this may be due to the reduced immune response in these patients. Chapter 12 by Kate Chadwick titled 'The importance of equity and accessibility: radiotherapy treatment for people with cancer and learning disability' discusses this important area in more detail.

Digestion

Poorer muscle tone can make digestions slower and more sluggish leading to greater absorption of water impacting on weight and also leading to constipation.

Dysphagia is the medical term for swallowing difficulties. Some people with dysphagia have problems swallowing certain foods or liquids, while others cannot swallow at all. Other signs of dysphagia include:

- coughing or choking when eating or drinking
- bringing food back up, sometimes through the nose
- a sensation that food is stuck in your throat or chest
- persistent drooling of saliva
- being unable to chew food properly
- a 'gurgly' wet sounding voice when eating or drinking
- Over time, dysphagia can also cause symptoms such as weight loss and repeated chest infections.

Dysphagia affects up to 8% of people with a learning disability, of which 40% will experience recurrent chest infections. Aspiration pneumonitis causes 3.4% of deaths and is potentially avoidable. The cause could be neurological or anatomical, secondary to a developmental abnormality (a structural abnormality of the mouth and throat). Assessment by a GP or speech and language therapist is normally the initial management. Public Health England (2016) has published guidelines on practical issues: https://www.gov.uk/government/publications/dysphagia-and-people-with-learning-disabilities. In this document you will find information about assessment, management, eating and drinking guidelines and medication.

Gastro-oesophageal reflux disease (GORD) affects 6.8% of patients with a learning disability. Those at higher risk are patients with cerebral palsy, scoliosis, or those being treated with anticonvulsants or long-term benzodiazepines. It can commonly affect sleep and behaviour and is a risk factor for oesophageal cancer. In reflux and GORD, the stomach contents and acid are expelled upwards from the stomach through the lower oesophageal sphincter into the oesophagus and mouth.

As asymmetrical body shape can affect the internal body systems, including compromising the stomach and digestive tract, it is important to look at providing smaller nutritional meals more often rather than attempting to give the person three large meals each day. Chapter 9 by Sarah Clayton and Anna Goldsmith titled 'Protection of body shape' discusses considerations for asymmetrical body shape and the importance of postural care in more detail.

Pain

> Pain is…what the experiencing person says it is, existing whenever he says it does.
> (McCaffery, 1968).

We all experience pain at times during our lives and know what action we should take when this happens. Self-reporting is recognised as the 'gold standard' for measuring pain as it is a subjective experience.

People with a learning disability may find it hard to tell someone that they are in pain due to communication difficulties and the severity of their learning disability. Yet they are also at increased risk of experiencing health conditions which may cause pain.

There is a misconception that people with learning disabilities have a higher pain tolerance than people who do not have a learning disability. Whilst some people do have impaired neural pathways others may have increased sensitivity to pain. Some people do not express pain in the conventional way; possibly hitting the side of their face to indicate dental pain or earache.

Pharmacology

Medications can resolve one problem and cause another as side effects, which can impact on vital signs. Be aware some medications may treat pain like codeine and cause problems like constipation.

Therefore, further medication or steps may need to be taken to minimise the side effects. Clear communication with patients about medications can help determine the extent of their unwanted side effects so they can be acted on.

References

BBC (2020) Coronavirus: pandemic sees spike in learning disabled deaths. Available at: https://www.bbc.co.uk/news/disability-52891401

Better Health (2021) Down syndrome and health. Available at: https://www.betterhealth.vic.gov.au/health/healthyliving/down-syndrome-and-health [Accessed 07.08.23]

Davis, S.R., Durvasula, S., Merhi, D., Young, P.M., Traini, D. and Bosnic-Anticevich, S Z. (2015) The role of direct support professionals in asthma management. *Journal of Intellectual & Developmental Disability*, 40(4): 342–353.

Delves-Yates, C. (2022) *Essentials of Nursing Practice*, 3rd edition. London: Sage Publications.

Folch, A., Salvador-Curulla, L., Vicens, P., Cortes, M.J., Irazebal, M., Munoz, S., Rovira, L., Orejula, C., Gonzalez, J.A. and Martinez-Leal, R. (2017) Health indicators in intellectual development disorders: the key findings of POMONA-ESP project. *Journal of Applied Research in Intellectual Disability*, 32: 23–34.

Lister, S., Hofland, J. and Grafton, H. (eds.) (2020, 10th edition) *The Royal Marsden Manual of Clinical Nursing Procedures*, Professional Edition. New York: John Wiley & Sons.

McCaffery, M. (1968) *Nursing Practice Theories Related to Cognition, Bodily Pain, and Man-Environment Interactions*. Los Angeles: University of California at LA Students Store.

NHS inform (2024) Down's syndrome. Available at: https://www.nhsinform.scot/illnesses-and-conditions/downs-syndrome#:~:text=Around%20half%20of%20all%20children,and%20types%20of%20heart%20disease. [Accessed 08.08.23]

NIH (National Institute of Child Health and Human Development) (2017) What conditions or disorders are commonly associated with Down syndrome? What conditions or disorders are commonly associated with Down syndrome? | NICHD - Eunice Kennedy Shriver National Institute of Child Health and Human Development (nih.gov) [Accessed 07.08.23]

Northway, R. and Hopes, P. (2022) *Learning Disability Nursing: Developing Professional Practice*. St Albans: Critical Publishing.

Resuscitation Council UK (2021) The ABCDE Approach [Online]. Resuscitation Council UK. Available at: https://www.resus.org.uk/library/abcde-approach [Accessed 21/10/23]

Royal College of Physicians (2017) National Early Warning Score (NEWS) 2. Available at: https://www.rcp.ac.uk/improving-care/resources/national-early-warning-score-news-2/ [Accessed 22.09.2023]

Page, A. and Wakeman, M. (2017) Considerations nurses caring for people with a learning disability should think about when undertaking nursing observations – a framework. *Learning Disability Practice*, 20(4): 18–19. https://rcni.com/learning-disability-practice/features/nurses-need-to-know-appropriate-clinical-range-when-taking-observations-88246

Prasher, V.P. and Janicki, M.P. (2002) *Physical Health of Adults with Intellectual Disabilities*. Oxford: Blackwell.

Public Health England (2016) Dysphagia and people with learning disabilities: guidance on providing support and reasonable adjustments to meet the needs of people with learning disabilities who have difficulty swallowing (dysphagia) https://www.gov.uk/government/publications/dysphagia-and-people-with-learning-disabilities [Accessed 21.9.2023]

Public Health England (2020) Eye care and people with learning disabilities: making reasonable adjustments. Available at: https://www.gov.uk/government/publications/eye-care-and-people-with-learning-disabilities/eye-care-and-people-with-learning-disabilities-making-reasonable-adjustments?fbclid=IwAR21Wm2I-sjjQtv5bWjozTrFkcGVqxdwo4dE0aKAVXe3iOOIIgWDjylX_s0 [Accessed 21.9.2023]

University of Hertfordshire Intellectual Disability and Health https://www.intellectualdisability.info/ [Accessed 21.9.2023]

Protection of body shape

Anna Goldsmith and Sarah Clayton

We hear the word 'posture' on a daily basis. Maybe you've joked about having bad posture when you sit at your desk at work, or you've tried to make improvements to your posture with an evening yoga class. We know that having good posture can help with alleviating back pain, neck pain and movement. However, posture goes far beyond this. Poor posture can have life-threatening complications for individuals at risk of body shape distortion (Carter, 2017). This chapter will take you through the concept of 'posture' as the blueprint for not only your physical health, but your mental health and overall quality of life.

'Posture' is defined by the *Oxford English Dictionary* as the 'position in which someone holds their body when standing or sitting'. In certain positions the body has to work harder to maintain its posture and at other times the body can be more relaxed; for example, when someone is standing compared to when someone is lying down. The skeletal system, a complex structure comprising bone, cartilage, ligaments and tendons, is encased within muscle and soft tissue. These muscles, tissues and ligaments work together to hold the body in certain positions. The effect of gravity on the body is depicted through weight, and gravity will pull down on these muscles and tissues no matter what position someone is in.

There are certain phrases which are important to understand from a posture perspective. Some will be used in this chapter. Here is a short glossary for your information:

Body shape distortion – destructive changes in someone's body shape

Supine lying – lying on your back

Side lying – lying on your side

Prone lying – lying on your tummy

Scoliosis – a sideways curve of the spine

Kyphosis – a forwards curve of the spine, usually at the top of the neck

Lordosis – a curve of the spine inwards at the lumbar (lower) part of the spine

Flexion – the action of 'bending', i.e. a bent joint such as a knee or a hip

DOI: 10.4324/9781003341765-11

Extension – the action of straightening, such as straightening a joint

Hip migration – the percentage to which the head of the femur (top of the leg bone) is starting to come out of the socket

Subluxation – when the head of the femur is coming out of the socket

Dislocation – when the head of the femur is completely out of the socket

Supported lying – when an individual is provided with positioning supports so the body is held gently in position

Unsupported – when an individual is left with no support so the body is left to fall into destructive positions

Wheelchair seating – a chair with wheels which enables a person who finds it harder to walk to get out and about

Alternative seating – usually a more comfortable chair which provides support for the person outside of their wheelchair

Manual chair – a wheelchair that is powered by either the person themselves or by someone pushing the chair

Powerchair – a wheelchair which is moved by using battery power

Tilt and recline – two features on a wheelchair which allow both the whole seat to be tilted backwards and for the backrest to recline

Standing frame – a device which allows a person to stand by using straps and supports to bring them upwards

Walking aids – a term to encompass anything which helps someone to walk. This might include walking sticks or frames

Gait trainer – a device that uses pelvic and trunk support to allow someone to walk with support

Sit to stand transfer – the movement of taking someone from sitting to standing. This might include using a device to make the movement easier.

What is positioning?

Positioning, when it comes to the body, is about ways in which someone's body is aligned. Positioning occurs in sitting, standing and lying. Some people can move themselves in and out of position more easily than others and so may not need as much help to adapt their position. However, if someone is unable to change position independently, they will be reliant on others to alter their position throughout the day and, sometimes, the night.

The issue with having an inability to change position can mean that an individual is left in a destructive position over time. The combined effect of a destructive position and the compressive effect of gravity on the body has been well documented to cause catastrophic changes in body shape (Fulford and Brown, 1976).

These changes in body shape have often been thought to be synonymous with having a complex disability but this is simply not the case. A number of the issues caused through a lack of support in the lying posture can not only be prevented but, excitingly, can also be reversed.

These destructive positions are known to cause problems such as those shown below and more:

- the musculoskeletal system (contractures, loss of joint integrity, for example hip dislocation, decreased bone density, reduced range of joint motion and deformity, such as spinal scoliosis)

- the neurological system (spasticity/muscle tone, primitive reflexes, altered sensation and joint position sense, pain, weakness)

- respiratory function

- digestion (including swallowing and choking, both of which are compromised by poor head and neck posture) and kidney/renal function

- personal hygiene, ease of [continence] and changing

- functional ability

- environment interaction (sensory perception, body aesthetics, learning, communication), sleep pattern and irritability.

(Hill and Goldsmith, 2010)

This insidious deterioration in body shape can often happen slowly, over a number of years, which can mean it is often not spotted before more serious consequences develop. It can also be more challenging for one particular healthcare professional or individual to be solely responsible for an individual's postural care as it clearly affects so many different facets of someone's life. Whilst it affects bodily structures, this isn't solely a physiotherapist's responsibility. Whilst it affects someone's ability to function, this isn't solely an occupational therapist's responsibility. Whilst this affects swallowing and digestion, this isn't solely a speech and language therapist's responsibility and so on and so on … posture and protection of body shape is everyone's responsibility.

FRED

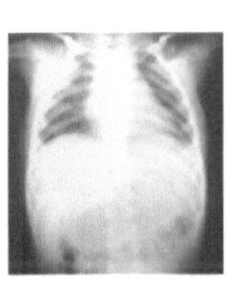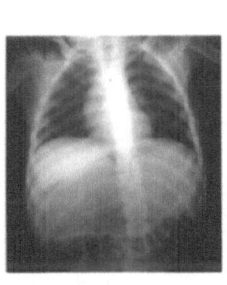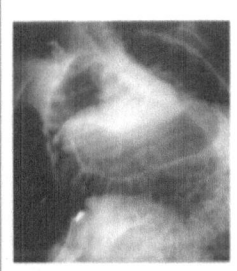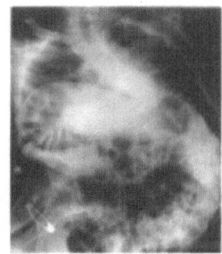

FIGURE 9.1 Protecting body shape – Fred (Pawlyn and Carnaby, 2008)

So, who could this affect?

Why are some people more at risk than others with regards to body shape distortion? We know that individuals with movement difficulties can find it harder to alter their position throughout the day and night which could leave them in destructive positions at the mercy of gravity. Therefore, anyone who has a movement problem should be supported to understand the impact of their position over a long period of time. For those people who are supported by carers the whole support team will need to understand the consequences of a lack of postural care.

It has been acknowledged that more complex body shapes can often be seen in those with more complex disability where movement is severely impacted. 'Postural deformity exhibiting complex aspects, such as scoliosis, windswept hip deformity, pelvic obliquity, and hip dislocation, is frequently seen in children with severe cerebral palsy, who can hardly move by themselves' (Sato, 2020). However, this model runs the risk of excluding less complicated individuals who may also be at risk of body shape distortion.

To fully investigate if someone is at risk of developing changes in their body shape there are a number of tools which can used. Thorough collaboration with an individual and their family to address a person's habitual postures is needed to understand what, if any, risks are posed. Tools such as the Mansfield checklist can be used to get an understanding of someone's preferred postures which can then be discussed:

1 Does the body stay in a limited number of positions?

2 Do the knees seem to be drawn usually to one side, or inwards, or outwards into a 'frog' posture?

3 Does the head seem to turn mainly to one side?

4 Does the body tend to flex forward, or extend backwards, or both?

5 Is the body shape already asymmetric?

(Hill, 2000)

Affirmative answers to any of the above questions would imply that someone could potentially be at risk of developing changes in their body shape and preventable, secondary complications.

Who do you need to involve?

Positioning brings with it a wide variety of risk for some individuals, and a collaborative approach with those closest to them will need to be used. The importance of engaging with, and utilising the knowledge of, the person in need of postural care and the individuals closest to them cannot be underestimated. Recent research into postural care services found that 'provision needs to move away from a medical model of providing equipment and episodic regimes of therapy. Rather, it must begin to function within a self-management model reliant upon the empowerment of families through coaching, co-ordination, and coproduction' (Wright and Clayton, 2020).

For a postural care plan to be successful this cannot be the remit of one individual. There are a multitude of concerns which need to be thought through which, in turn, will bring in the requirement for another person's input. Firstly, postural care for someone who is at risk of body shape distortion will need to be looked at over the whole 24-hour period. Essentially, it is key to understand that in all postures, at all times of the day and throughout someone's entire life, gravity will be impacting on the body.

Depending on the age of the person and where they spend their days you may require involvement from:

- Teachers
- Physiotherapists
- Occupational therapists (OT)
- Speech and language therapy
- Nurses
- Colleagues
- Personal assistants
- Day-centre staff

Throughout the day someone may need to be seated in order to get to work, school, activities and events. This may require the need for a variety of seating options which will not only maximise someone's postural care but will also allow them to function well and enjoy their life. For example, one person's seating may be different to another's as their vision or communication needs will differ. One person may need access to a communication aid such as an eye gaze, whilst someone else may be self-propelling their wheelchair. Some people may also need to have access to alternative positions for rest and other health-related needs such as postural drainage.

Once an individual's daytime positioning has been successfully considered then the rest of the 24-hour period needs to addressed too. After all, gravity doesn't turn off at night-time!

At night-time some people, if they aren't supported by night staff, are less monitored and therefore more vulnerable than during the day. A full safety checklist should be considered when addressing someone's postural care needs at night, taking in to account issues such as:

- Continence
- Breathing (use of oxygen saturation monitors can be helpful when making changes to someone's position)
- Secretion management
- Temperature regulation

- ■ Seizure activity

- ■ Pressure care

This list is not exhaustive.

Case study

Samara is 14 years old. She does not communicate using words but people who know her will say that this is no barrier to her letting you know what she wants, needs, likes and dislikes! She can be very clear on these things! Samara is able to walk short distances around her home and garden. When she is out and about she uses a manual wheelchair which she is able to self-propel although her family say that she is finding this more difficult. Samara has a fantastic social network and is an active member at her local leisure centre. She loves to swim, to go to aquarobics and meet her friends for a cup of tea.

Over the last six months there has been a significant deterioration in Samara's mental health. She is usually described as outgoing, fun loving and sociable but recently she has become withdrawn. She doesn't seem to want to go out as often and when she is out for longer than an hour she becomes distressed and indicates that she wants to go home. Her family say that her bottom has started sliding forward in her wheelchair and that her feet keep falling off the front of her footplates. She indicates that she is uncomfortable and there are concerns that she is in pain after time in her wheelchair. Samara is becoming isolated from her friends, she is putting on weight as she is less active and is struggling to manage her emotions, becoming short-tempered and tearful.

Think Point

Do you think the chair is currently suitable?

Which other healthcare professionals could you ask for support?

Where might you find further information about the chair and Samara's seating needs? Remember to consider informal information from involving family members.

How would you escalate a concern?

What would be the impact of using a chair that is uncomfortable?

How would an uncomfortable chair impact on a person's mental health? Their physical health? Their skin? Their ability to maintain an active social life?

There are a variety of different outcomes here for Samara based on a multitude of factors. We are going to consider two.

Outcome 1

- ■ Samara's family approaches her occupational therapist about her seating and tell him their concerns.

- The OT refers Samara back to wheelchair services to see if there is anything to be done about her comfort in the wheelchair. It is a long wait for her to be seen by them.

- During the wait Samara deteriorates further and starts to get regular chest infections. She is hospitalised for two weeks during which she develops a pressure injury on her sacrum. When she is finally discharged from hospital she can no longer sit in her wheelchair at all, leaving her confined to her bed.

- Samara's positioning in bed is dictated by her pressure injury so she can only lie on one side. She begins to develop a strong kyphosis and progressive flexion of her hips and knees leading to the development of contractures.

- Samara's mum and dad can no longer take care of Samara's needs alone. Her manual handling requirements are too complex, leading to a care agency being commissioned to support her.

- Samara's dad is very distressed by the lack of involvement he can now have in his daughter's care and becomes depressed.

- The entire family become isolated from their community, Samara becomes more and more withdrawn resulting in the need for antidepressant medication alongside an increase in pain medication for her.

- Samara's body shape changes to such an extent that she can no longer find any comfortable position. The changes in Samara's body shape begin to impact on her health further, she suffers from debilitating constipation, repeated chest infections and has difficulty breathing…eventually her body shape becomes no longer compatible with living and Samara dies aged 16 from pneumonia.

Outcome 2

- Samara's family approaches her occupational therapist about her seating and tell him their concerns.

- The OT refers Samara back to wheelchair services to see if there is anything to be done about her comfort in the wheelchair. It is a long wait for her to be seen by them.

- As it is such a long wait, the OT calls on his physiotherapy colleagues to see if anything can be done to maximise Samara's posture at other times during the day.

- The physios and OT work together to develop a lying posture plan for Samara.

- Samara's teachers and her teaching assistants work with the therapy team to find times during the day when Samara can be out of her wheelchair and her body shape maximised in the lying posture.

- They make use of equipment such as her standing frame and positioning system so she can enjoy her education in a variety of different positions.

- As Samara is really enjoying these opportunities for therapy in the lying posture during the day the therapy team ask her family if they want to look at using the same therapy at home too.

- Samara begins to be positioned in a supported position at home while she watches her evening film with her siblings. Over time she becomes so used to this routine she falls asleep in her supported position and wakes up feeling refreshed and relaxed.

- Samara's body shape is supported and not allowed to deteriorate during the wait for her wheelchair appointment.

- When the time comes to look at her new chair it is found that she has grown by a full 3 inches and that the old seating system doesn't fit her anymore.

- Alongside with understanding how her lying posture therapy is making such a positive difference to her health and wellbeing, her seating could mirror this and also maximise her function during the day.

- Samara is soon back to exploring her world with her friends, enjoying her swimming, and her family are thrilled to have the old, happy Samara back again!

Useful links

Simple Stuff works – a family-run organisation offering world-leading training advice and equipment around posture: www.simplestuffworks.com

Changing Our Lives is a rights-based organisation working to make an ordinary life possible for disabled people: https://changingourlives.org/wp-content/uploads/2023/12/Postural-Care-Overview-MASTER.pdf

PAMIS is a Scottish organisation that works with people with a profound and multiple learning disability and their families for a better life: https://pamis.org.uk/services/postural-care/

Measurement of body symmetry videos – developed by Simple Stuff Works: https://youtube.com/playlist?list=PLx7Dyp1wZw_tG6pwR4PVMMHmIYHd2PAD7&si=LI6_38SOhbLg-CyR (Measurement of Body Symmetry Videos)

References

Carter, B. (2017) *Poor posture in people with disabilities can be fatal*. https://theconversation.com/poor-posture-in-people-with-disabilities-can-be-fatal-86251 (accessed December 2023).

Fulford, G.E. and Brown, J.K. (1976) 'Position as a cause of deformity in children with Cerebral Palsy', *Developmental Medicine & Child Neurology*, 18, 305–314.

Goldsmith, S. (2000) 'The Mansfield project: postural care at night within a community setting: a feedback study', *Physiotherapy*, 86, 10, 528–534.

Hill, S. and Goldsmith, E. (2008) 'Posture, mobility and comfort', in J. Pawlyn and S. Carnaby (eds), *Profound Intellectual and Multiple Disabilities*, 328–347.

Hill, S. and Goldsmith, J. (2010) 'Biomechanics and prevention of body shape distortion', *The Tizard Learning Disability Review*, 15, 2, 15–29.

Sato, H. (2020) Postural deformity in children with cerebral palsy: Why it occurs and how is it managed, *Physical Therapy Research*, 23, 1, pp 8–14.

Wright, R. and Clayton, S. (2020) *Posture Positive: Postural Care in the Age of Covid19*. Available at: Posture-Positive-Summary-2.pdf (bornattherighttime.com)

10

Considerations for delivery of cardiopulmonary resuscitation (CPR) and choking management to people with profound and multiple learning disability and wheelchair users

Elisha Deegan, Andrea Page and Stefan Cash

Background

Nurses the world over are frequently first responders to in-hospital arrests and as such are expected to learn and refresh their skills in delivery of cardiopulmonary resuscitation (CPR) and other emergency care regularly (Moon et al., 2020; Sok et al., 2020; Rikhotso et al., 2021). Nursing students together with other health-care students are considered experts in management of emergency situations by the general public; however, research demonstrates that their knowledge and skills often do not comply with resuscitation council guidelines (Kim and Roh, 2016; Demirtas et al., 2021). Simulation-based education that is delivered as frequently as six-monthly is effective in improving students' confidence, knowledge and performance during CPR (Kim & Roh, 2016; Demirtas et al., 2021; Rikhotso et al., 2021). For specific and specialist populations, such as people who are pregnant, have had a drug overdose, been caught in an avalanche or who have asthma, that require care in addition to the standard care, resuscitation councils have developed supplemental guidelines (ANZCOR, 2011; Cimpoesu et al., 2019). For nurses working in the disability sector there are no supplemental guidelines or evidence-based educational interventions for delivery of CPR or basic life support (BLS) to people with disabilities (Page & Cash, 2011; Thomas, 2020; Deegan et al., 2022). This lack of specific guidance leaves nurses, healthcare professionals and disability support staff in a position where they are having to adjust standard care to meet the needs of people with disabilities during emergency situations, resulting in increased delays until care is initiated and an increase in premature or

DOI: 10.4324/9781003341765-12

preventable deaths (Heslop et al., 2013; Heslop et al., 2019; Trollor and Salomon, 2019a; Royal Mencap Society, 2022).

The scale of the problem for people with disabilities

People with disabilities make up approximately 16% of the worldwide population, which equates to one in six people (World Health Organization (WHO), 2018). Definitions for profound or complex disability are not universal, but this term generally relates to people whose disabilities mean they require assistance with many activities of daily living, as well as communication, and are most likely to have a learning or intellectual disability together with physical disabilities (Australian Institute of Health and Welfare, 2022; Sense, 2023). There are approximately 1.5 million people with complex or profound disabilities in both the UK and Australia, so whilst this population is a minority there are significant numbers of people living with profound and complex disabilities (Australian Institute of Health and Welfare, 2022; Sense, 2023). People with profound or complex disabilities have an increased likelihood of having body shape distortions due to limited or restricted movements, which can result in atypical chest shape (Hill and Goldsmith, 2010; Clayton and Ellis, 2015). There are also many people with disabilities who use wheelchairs. Body distortions and wheelchair use have been identified as creating challenges during the delivery of CPR and BLS, which includes choking recognition and management (Page and Cash, 2011; Deegan et al., 2022). Delivery of CPR and BLS to people with distorted body shapes and wheelchair users has previously been identified by Learning Disability nursing students in the UK as being one of their most feared clinical situations (Page and Cash, 2011).

Inequality of care

There are vast amounts of literature and evidence that highlight the disparities in healthcare that exist for people with disability. The inequality of care received by people with disability generally increases proportionately alongside the impact of the person's disability, meaning people with profound and multiple disability are the people who experience the most difficulty accessing optimal healthcare (Mencap, 2004, 2007, 2012; Mansell, 2010; Heslop et al., 2013; Heslop et al., 2019; Trollor and Salomon, 2019a).

Unequal access to healthcare for people with disability contributes to premature and preventable deaths, which are significantly more prevalent for people with disability than for people without disability. The prevalence of preventable and premature deaths has been documented by many organisations and governing bodies internationally for over a decade (Mencap, 2012; Heslop et al., 2019; Trollor and Salomon, 2019a). Furthermore it has been highlighted by these organisations that there is a large difference in life expectancy for people with disability compared to people without disability. The Learning Disability Mortality Review by Heslop et al. (2019) reports this gap to be 23 years for males and 27 years for females.

Examination and reporting of the deaths that occur in the disability population is completed regularly to identify areas for improvement and provide recommendations for service providers to reduce preventable and premature deaths. Throughout these reports one of the recommendations that has been posed many times is the improvement of first aid responses by care providers, including an improvement in the early recognition of signs that indicate deteriorating health (Heslop et al., 2013; Heslop et al., 2019; Trollor and Salomon, 2019b). This is a recommendation that has been made for more than a decade across the world, yet care givers, healthcare staff and nurses still do not have access to disability specific guidelines for delivery of first aid, CPR or basic life support which includes choking management (Page and Cash, 2011; Thomas, 2020; Deegan et al., 2023).

Ideas to supplement standard care

In the UK, Safety, Stimulate/Shake and Shout (SSS) followed by Airway, Breathing, Circulation, Defibrillation, Exposure (ABCDE) is used as mnemonic to recall the sequential steps of delivering BLS (Resuscitation Council UK, 2021a)

Using this mnemonic as a framework a number of considerations for augmentation are posed in Table 10.1.

TABLE 10.1 Basic life support considerations for an adult

	Extracts taken from Resuscitation Council UK guidelines (2021)	Considerations to take into account the person's disability
Safety	Ensure it is safe to approach	Ensure safety of any other people with a disability in your care and the safety of colleagues within this situation. Safety includes equipment used by individuals such as feeding pumps which could be a trip hazard. Be aware that this situation may lead to distressed behaviours (behaviours of concern) in others which may also have to be managed during this time.
Stimulate/ **S**hake	Gently shake the person's shoulder, arms or legs, looking for any response and signs of life. Ask if they are ok.	Is the person able to respond verbally? What response will alert you to the person's consciousness? What response is typical for this person? Perhaps ask them to open their eyes or squeeze your hand as a response rather than relying on a verbal response.
Shout	Shout for help and the local guidelines and procedures. This could include calling for an ambulance or making an internal alert call	In shouting for help consider what kind of extra assistance you may need? Do you need a number of people to assist with moving the person? Do you need equipment brought to you? For example, when you call for an ambulance remember to let them know the person has a disability or is in a wheelchair so that the paramedics can prepare for the situation.

(Continued)

TABLE 10.1 (*Continued*)

	Extracts taken from Resuscitation Council UK guidelines (2021)	Considerations to take into account the person's disability
Airway	Open the airway with a head tilt/chin lift manoeuvre.	Have you risk assessed how to maintain the airway for this person? Are you aware of a specific care plan highlighting this (i.e. BLS risk assessment or a postural management care plan one? Can you tilt the person's head? If not, have you been taught how to administer a jaw thrust? Have you been taught how to use an airway adjunct (e.g. naso pharyngeal airway or oral pharyngeal airway)? Is the person in a wheelchair? If yes, how does this impact on maintaining their airway and the actions you now have to take? If the person is in a wheelchair or has limited neck movement through a spinal fusion or muscular contractions which makes maintaining the airway difficult, a jaw thrust may be easier to maintain than a head tilt. NB: If the person has a percutaneous endoscopic gastrostomy (PEG) feed running stop this to reduce chance of aspiration or vomiting. NB: If there is suction equipment available and you have received appropriate training, consider using it to deliver oropharyngeal suction.
Breathing	Look for signs of life. This includes look, listen and feel for breaths for 10 seconds	What is 'normal' breathing for this person? Are there any changes to their breathing sounds that are not typical for them? NB: Also consider if they have an atypical chest shape that the rise and fall of the chest may not be symmetrical or may be difficult to observe.
	If the person is unconscious but breathing normally place them in the recovery position and maintain an open and clear airway.	Maintaining an open and clear airway may be easier with a jaw thrust. If the person is in a wheelchair, you may be able to maintain a clear and open airway while they remain seated; however, you must remain vigilant to any signs of choking, vomiting or regurgitation so that you can turn the person's head to the side quickly and clear the airway as needed. Alternatively, you could hold the head to the side whilst maintaining a jaw thrust.
	If the person is unconscious and not breathing normally prepare to deliver CPR.	If the person is in a wheelchair and you have enough help move the person to a hard flat surface.

(*Continued*)

TABLE 10.1 (*Continued*)

	Extracts taken from Resuscitation Council UK guidelines (2021)	Considerations to take into account the person's disability
Circulation	CPR should be delivered at a ratio of 30 compressions to 2 breaths for an adult. Compressions are delivered on the lower half of the sternum (in the centre of the chest) to a depth of 5–6 cm and at a rate of 100–120 per minute.Breaths	If the person is in a wheelchair which can 'tilt in space' and you have not been able to move them to the floor, consider tilting the wheelchair to lay the person as flat as possible and commence compressions in this position until the person can be moved. If the person is in a wheelchair that cannot be tilted, consider using the techniques described for removing a person from a chair in the Guidance for Safer Handling during resuscitation in healthcare settings (Pitcher, 2013), to move them to the ground as safely as possible. Tipping the wheelchair is not recommended due to the risk of injury to the rescuer and the person.
	As part of this process, once you have completed 30 chest compressions, if available, use a bag and valve mask (BVM), attached to oxygen, to deliver the two ventilations (breaths), alternatively in the community a pocket mask can be used. Continue with this process until the person recovers, help arrives or you physically are unable to continue any more.	If the person has an atypical chest shape be aware that the sternum may not be in the centre of the chest. Feel for the top (sternal notch) and bottom (xiphoid process) of the sternum to assess where the sternum is situated and place hands on the lower half. If there is a need for airway adjunct or the delivery of a jaw thrust to maintain an open airway, delivery of rescue breaths will be easier if using a bag and valve mask or a pocket mask. Consider having this equipment available and receiving the necessary training to use this equipment.
Defibrillation	Attach a defibrillator when it becomes available and follow all prompts given by the machine.	If the person has an atypical chest shape consider the positioning of the defibrillator pads to ensure that they are situated with the heart lying between them. If the person is particularly small or frail and pad placement on the chest wall is difficult consider placing one pad on the front of the chest and the other on the back of the chest.
Choking	Suspect choking if the person is suddenly unable to speak or talk, particularly if eating. Conscious – encourage the person to cough; if the cough is or becomes ineffective commence with 5 back blows followed by 5 abdominal thrusts. Unconscious – Start CPR. (Resuscitation Council UK, 2021b)	People with a learning or physical disability and an altered body shape may start choking for a variety of reasons including (Page and Cash, 2011): • Eating • Issues with swallowing • Excess secretions • Immature or inhibited gag reflex • Position in a wheelchair • Placing objects in their mouth • Vomiting Anything that could cause choking should be reviewed to minimise risk. Knowing the individual and understanding what position they need to be in during certain activities, such as eating, will ensure the risk of choking is minimised (Page and Cash, 2011). If the person is seated in a wheelchair and abdominal thrusts are not achievable continue with back blows. If the person is unconscious, see above for delivery of CPR.

Please note, these considerations are developed from expert opinion and should only be used in the event that the standard guidelines cannot be applied. All CPR and BLS should be delivered as close as possible to the UK Resuscitation Council Guidelines (2021).

Recommendation for improvement

Research to demonstrate the clinical effectiveness of techniques suggested in the table are ongoing. However, there has been a small intervention study that demonstrated that delivery of the suggestions in the table to carers of people with disability has significantly increased their confidence to act in scenarios that included people with disability. Furthermore, the increased confidence to act was retained by carers over a six-month period (Deegan et al., 2022).

Due to the alarming rates of deaths caused by choking and subsequent aspiration pneumonia (Heslop et al., 2019; Trollor and Salomon, 2019a) it is recommended that choking management, recognition and choking care is included in annual CPR updates for all carers and healthcare professionals providing care to people with disability.

The current situation

There are currently minimal guidelines available for carers and healthcare workers that inform how to deliver CPR/BLS to people with disability. Care givers are often left to determine the best way to augment standard guidelines individually and this creates fear and anxiety about these scenarios.

It has been well established over more than a decade that people with disability are dying premature and preventable deaths and one of the recognised causes is poor access to optimal healthcare for people with disability. Recommendations from mortality reports on people with disability have consistently included improved CPR/BLS training for carers and healthcare professionals on how to recognise and treat emerging illness in people with disability.

Inclusion of ideas for how to supplement standard CPR/BLS for delivery to people with disability has demonstrated increased confidence to act which leads to improved willingness to act. In the absence of further research to demonstrate clinical effectiveness it is reasonable to use expert opinion to inform the delivery of CPR/BLS where the standard care is not achievable.

References

Anzcor 2011. Guideline 11.10 Resuscitation in special circumstances [Online]. Australian Resuscitation Council. Available: https://resus.org.au/guidelines/ [Accessed 26/5/2019].

Australian Institute of Health and Welfare 2022. People with disability in Australia. In AIHW (ed.) Catalogue number DIS 72 ed.

Cimpoesu, D., Corlade-Andrei, M., Popa, T. O., Grigorasi, G., Bouros, C., Rotaru, L. & Nedelea, P. L. 2019. Cardiac arrest in special circumstances—recent advances in resuscitation. *American Journal of Therapeutics*, 26, e276–e283.

Clayton, S. & Ellis, T. 2015. Shaping the future. *Learning Disability Today*, Nov/Dec, 16–17.

Deegan, E. M., Saunders, A., Wilson, N. J. & Mccann, D. 2022. Cardio-pulmonary-resuscitation for people who use a wheelchair and/or have an atypical chest shape: an educational intervention. *Disability and Rehabilitation*, 45(2), 1–8.

Deegan, E., Wilson, N. J., Pullin, L. H. & Lewis, P. 2023. Cardiopulmonary resuscitation and basic life support for people with atypical chest shapes and wheelchair users: Toward supplemented education and emergency management plans. *Disability and Health Journal*, 101501.

Demirtas, A., Guvenc, G., Aslan, Ö., Unver, V., Basak, T. & Kaya, C. 2021. Effectiveness of simulation-based cardiopulmonary resuscitation training programs on fourth-year nursing students. *Australasian Emergency Care*, 24, 4–10.

Heslop, Blair, Felming, Hoghton, Marriott & Russ 2013. Confidential Inquiry into Premature Deaths of People with Learning Disabilities (CIPOLD). University of Bristol.

Heslop, Calkin & Huxor 2019. The Learning Disability Mortality Review (LeDeR) Programme: Annual Report. University of Bristol Norah Fry Centre for Disability Studies.

Hill, S. & Goldsmith, J. 2010. Biomechanics and prevention of body shape distortion. *Tizard Learning Disability Review*, 15, 15–29.

Kim, S. S. & Roh, Y. S. 2016. Status of cardiopulmonary resuscitation curricula for nursing students: A questionnaire study. *Nursing & Health Sciences*, 18, 496–502.

Mansell, J. 2010. Raising our sights; services for adults with profound intellectual and multiple disabilities. Kent: Tizard Centre.

Mencap 2004. *Treat Me Right*. London: Mencap.

Mencap 2007. *Death by Indifference*. London: Mencap.

Mencap 2012. *Death by Indifference: 74 Deaths and Counting*. London: Mencap.

Moon, S., Ryoo, H. W., Ahn, J. Y., Lee, D. E., Shin, S. D. & Park, J. H. 2020. Association of response time interval with neurological outcomes after out-of-hospital cardiac arrest according to bystander CPR. *The American Journal of Emergency Medicine*, 38, 1760–1766.

Page, A. & Cash, S. 2011. Basic life support for people with profound and multiple learning disabilities. *Learning Disability Practice*, 14, 28–30.

Pitcher, D. (ed.) 2013. *Guidance for Safer Handing During Resuscitation in Healthcare Settings*. London.

Resuscitation Council UK. 2021a. *The ABCDE Approach* [Online]. Resuscitation Council UK. Available: https://www.resus.org.uk/library/abcde-approach [Accessed 21/10/23].

Resuscitation Council UK. 2021b. *Adult Choking* [Online]. Available: https://www.resus.org.uk/sites/default/files/2021-04/Adult%20Choking%20Algorithm%202021.pdf [Accessed 30/03/2023].

Rikhotso, M., Perrie, H., Scribante, J. & Jooma, Z. 2021. Cardiopulmonary resuscitation skills profile and knowledge of nurses working in an academic hospital. *SA Heart*, 18, 40–46.

Royal Mencap Society 2022. Annual Review. London: Mencap.

Sense. 2023. Complex disabilities [Online]. Sense. Available: https://www.sense.org.uk/information-and-advice/conditions/what-does-complex-disabilities-mean [Accessed 15/9/2023].

Sok, S. R., Kim, J. A., Lee, Y. & Cho, Y. 2020. Effects of a simulation-based CPR training program on knowledge, performance, and stress in clinical nurses. *The Journal of Continuing Education in Nursing*, 51, 225–232.

Thomas, C. 2020. Basic life support for children and young people with a learning or physical disability and an altered body shape. *Nursing Children and Young People*, 32, 24–31.

Trollor, J. & Salomon, C. 2019a. A scoping review of causes and contributors to deaths of people with disability in Australia. Sydney: University of New South Wales.

Trollor, J. & Salomon, C. 2019b. A scoping review of causes and contributors to deaths of people with disability in Australia, Summery of Recommendations. Sydney: University of New South Wales.

World Health Organization (WHO). 2018. *Disability and Health* [Online]. World Health Organization. Available: https://www.who.int/en/news-room/fact-sheets/detail/disability-and-health [Accessed 23/4/2019].

Clinical holding

Andrea Page, Alison Warren and Helen Jones

What is clinical holding?

This means using limited force to hold the patient still. Healthcare staff routinely use clinical holding to help infants, children, young people or adults stay still when treatment is being administered, to prevent them from interfering with the treatment, or when invasive examinations are being carried out (Page, Warren & Vanes, 2017).

What is the issue?

Healthcare staff rarely have any formal discussion with children, young people and adults, or their parents and carers, on the techniques used for clinical holding. Visual tools are important when talking to people with learning disabilities about their healthcare (Page, Warren & Vanes, 2017). A website with images of clinical holds would allow parents and carers to be able discuss relevant holds with their patients.

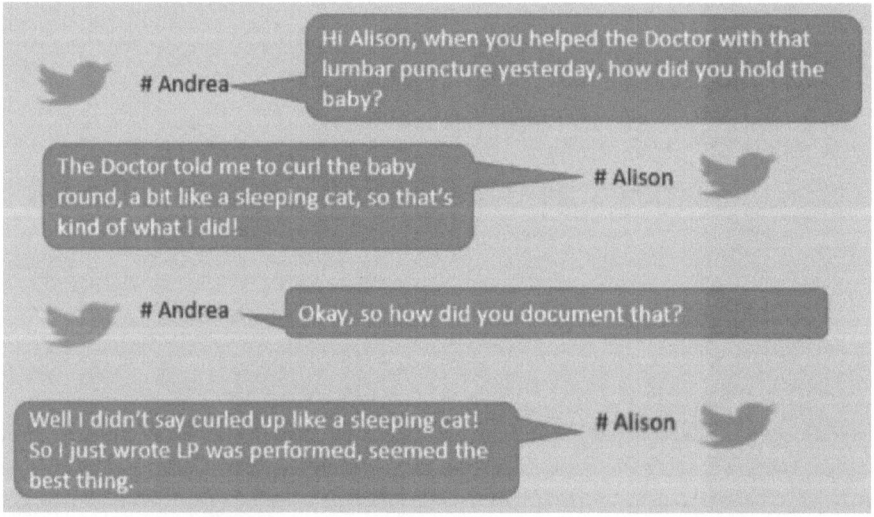

FIGURE 11.1 Andrea Alison tweet

DOI: 10.4324/9781003341765-13

Many people with a learning disability diagnosed with life-limiting conditions may display behaviours of concern when receiving medical care from healthcare professionals (Page et al., 2015). Therefore they are also at risk of being denied access to inpatient, acute and emergency care treatments, because healthcare staff are fearful of how to treat and care for them and believe no suitable support resources or facilities are available (Page et al., 2015). This can lead to poorer quality of life, ongoing health problems (Page and McDonnell, 2013) and diagnostic overshadowing.

The level of distress caused by a procedure should be an important consideration. The person may become distressed and as a result could even display behaviours viewed as aggressive. These behaviours can hinder the ability to perform a procedure safely, thus increasing anxiety (Page et al., 2019).

Where the use of restrictive physical interventions or clinical holding of children, young people and adults with a learning disability is concerned, healthcare staff must consider the rights of the person and the legal frameworks, including the Human Rights Act (1998), Mental Capacity Act (2005), the European Conventions on the Rights of the Child, Consent and Capacity Assessment (UN Convention on the Rights of the Child) (1989) and the Royal College of Nursing guidance (2019).

The RCN's (2019) 'Restrictive physical interventions and the clinical holding of children and young people: Clinical professional guidance' states:

■   Give careful consideration of whether the procedure is really necessary, and whether urgency in a situation prohibits the exploration of alternatives to holding.

What does this mean? How can/do you currently evidence this? Who decides?

■   Pause prior to a procedure to discuss and agree with a child and their parents/guardians what will happen during a procedure, what people's roles will be and if necessary what holding methods will be used, when they will be used and for how long.

What does this mean? How can/do you currently evidence this? Who decides?

■   Ensure that any holding used is the least restrictive option to meet the need and is used for the minimum amount of time. Nurses should make skilled use of minimum pressure and other age-appropriate techniques, such as wrapping and splinting.

What do they mean by skill use of maximum pressure? How can/do you currently evidence this? Who decides?

NB: The principles outlined above are also mentioned in relation to adults with a learning disability within the legal framework of the Mental Capacity Act (2005). Healthcare staff need to have received appropriate training around the Mental Capacity Act to inform their practice.

■   There must be a sufficient number of staff who are appropriately trained and confident in the process.

What kind of training do they mean? How can/do you currently evidence this? Who decides?

■ Ensure that any use of holding is fully and clearly documented in the child's plan of care and notes. (Accurate record keeping is essential – this should include why the intervention was necessary and details of what it involved.)

How can/do you currently evidence this? Who decides?

What can be done?

We imagine that you may have been struggling to answer the questions in italics. Why don't you put the following link into your browser and have a look at the sections and ideas on this website: https://chg.osimebcu.co.uk

How to use this site

■ Access the three main sections of the site by clicking on any of the images

■ We recommend that you look at the joints, movement and holding section first, then the clinical holds tool and finally the framework for clinical holding.

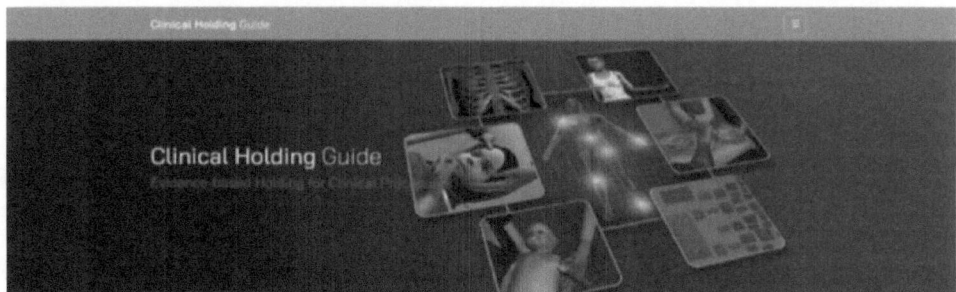

FIGURE 11.2 Clinical holding guide

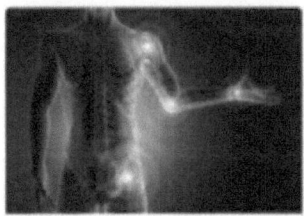 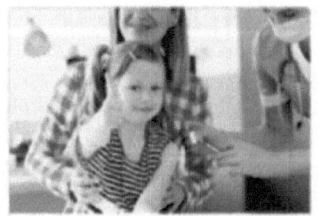 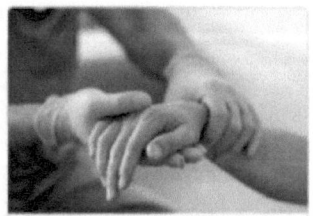

Joints, movement & holding
Have you ever thought about how the body moves? This section explains the different kinds of joints within the body, their range of movement and the consequences for clinical holding.

Clinical holds tool
This section illustrates various ways to hold a child in the event that it is necessary for them to undergo a specific clinical procedure. The procedure may require a child to be held still or to adopt a certain physical posture.

Framework for Clinical Holding
We recognise that there may be procedures which require a bespoke hold or which are not documented within this site. This framework has been developed to accommodate additional holds allowing the rationale and risks to be explored.

FIGURE 11.3 How to use site

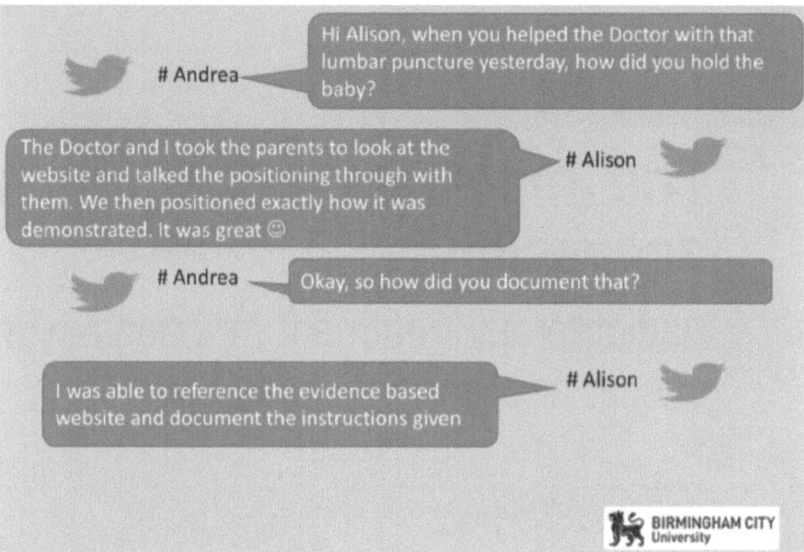

FIGURE 11.4 Andrea and Alison tweet evidence

Going back to all the questions in italics, this framework is written in such a way that it helps you consider all of these principles and there are two examples to guide you.

Useful resources and links

Clinical Holding Guide: https://chg.osimebcu.co.uk/(This resource could also be used in preparing the child for the procedure and could enhance the consent process)

Autism Speaks Autism Treatment Network: http://www.autismspeaks.org/sites/default/files/documents/atn/blood-draw-provider.pdf

Public Health England, 'Blood tests for people with learning disabilities: making reasonable adjustments': https://www.ndti.org.uk/assets/files/Blood_tests_for_people_with_learning_disabilities.pdf

References

Page, A., Elven, B., McDonnell, A, A., Warren, A., Vanes, N. and Seabra, S. (2019) Holding children and young people for procedures: ethical guidance for healthcare practitioners *Journal of Nursing Children and Young People*, 31(4): 28–33.

Page, A. & McDonnell, A, A. (2015) Holding children and young people: identifying a theory practice gap. *British Journal of Nursing*, 24(8): 378–382.

Page, A., Warren, A. and Vanes, N. (2017) Clinical holding an evaluation of a website developed through a collaboration between Birmingham City University and Birmingham Children's Hospital NHSFT. *Nursing Children and Young People*, 29(2); 20–24.

Royal College of Nursing (2019) Restrictive physical interventions and the clinical holding of children and young people: Clinical Professional Guidance. https://www.rcn.org.uk/-/media/royal-college-of-nursing/documents/publications/2019/october/007-746.pdf

12

The importance of equity and accessibility

Radiotherapy treatment for people with cancer and learning disability

Kate Chadwick

The bigger picture

Global rates of cancer are increasing dramatically with 24 million cases per year expected by 2035, a rise of 10 million since 2012 (Spencer et al., 2019). The mainstay cancer treatments widely available in the NHS include surgery, chemotherapy, other drug therapies and radiotherapy. Whilst surgery and chemotherapy are familiar amongst healthcare professionals and the general public alike, radiotherapy has remained the more mysterious and misunderstood cancer treatment. However, radiotherapy is used as a treatment option in half of all people with cancer and is a highly cost-effective treatment, contributing to around 40% of curative treatment (Baskar et al., 2012; Goodman, 2013; Duffton et al., 2020). It is therefore highly likely you will have individuals with learning disability and a cancer diagnosis who may benefit from radiotherapy treatment.

Radiotherapy is the treatment of cancerous tumours (and occasionally benign conditions) by the use of high energy, targeted radiation. Radiotherapy can be delivered both externally and internally by therapeutic radiographers. This chapter will focus on the more commonly used external beam radiotherapy where high energy X-rays are targeted at a tumour from outside the body by treatment machines called 'linear accelerators' or 'linacs' (see Figure 12.1). Due to recent advances in treatment technique, radiotherapy is now highly conformal, allowing treatment of tumours to very high doses with minimal effects on the surrounding tissues and 'organs at risk' (OAR), those tissues deemed to be at risk of permanent damage from radiation overdose (Symonds et al., 2012; Duffton et al., 2020). For this reason, radiotherapy is now a far more tolerable and manageable treatment than many people believe.

DOI: 10.4324/9781003341765-14

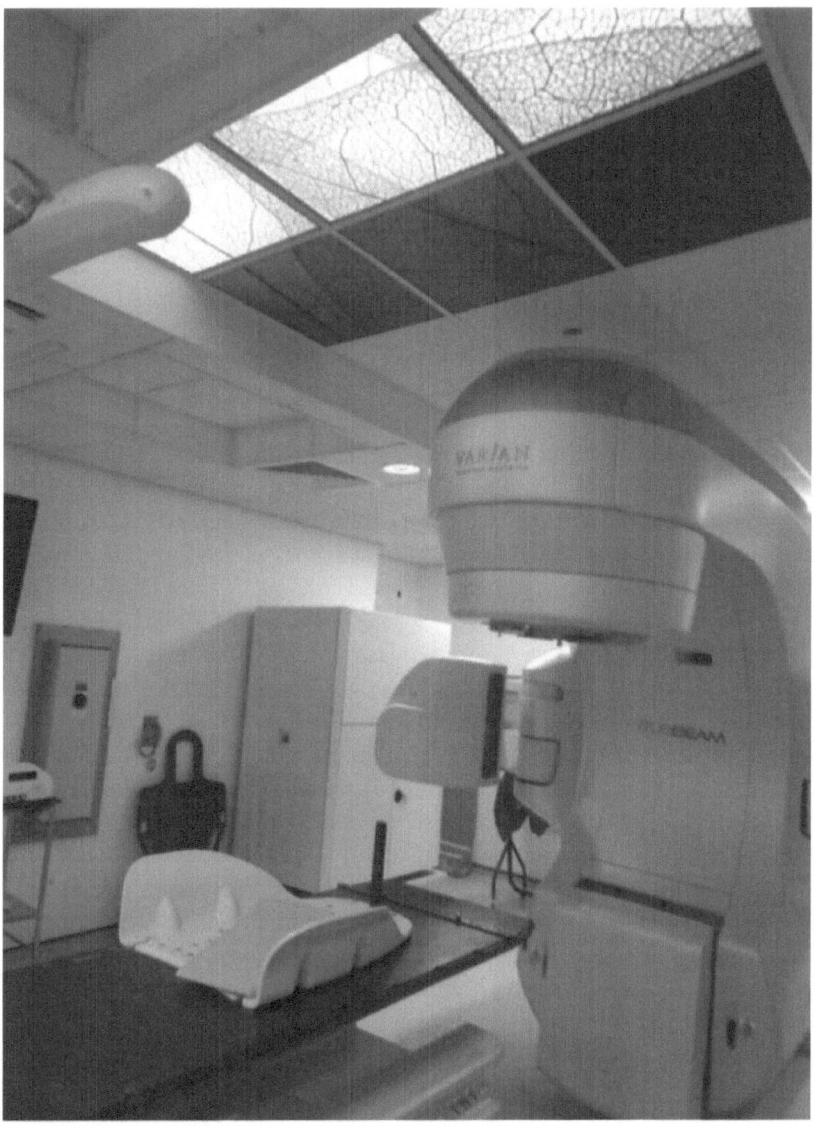

FIGURE 12.1 A linear accelerator radiotherapy treatment machine

Why is demystifying radiotherapy treatment important for healthcare professionals caring for people with a learning disability?

Epidemiological studies in Finland and Australia have shown that there is very little difference between the numbers of people developing cancer who have a learning disability and the general population (Sullivan et al., 2004; Patja et al., 2001). People with a learning disability are living longer, and with cancer being more prevalent in older age groups, the number of people with cancer and a learning disability presenting for radiotherapy treatment should be increasing (Tuffrey-Wijne, 2010). Yet despite this, and increasing cancer rates globally, numbers of individuals with a learning disability accessing radiotherapy are very low. There is a paucity of published information on the reasons for this specifically within therapeutic radiography, though it is known that institutional discrimination towards individuals with a learning disability occurs throughout the NHS, leading to a failure to attend healthcare settings, misdiagnosis, lack of appropriate care and diagnostic overshadowing (Mencap, 2007, 2012; Parliamentary and Health Service Ombudsman, 2009; Heslop et al., 2013).

National media frequently reports on the inequity of healthcare provision for individuals with a learning disability (Holt, 2017; Wood, 2018) and the Learning Disability Mortality Review (LeDeR) Programme Annual Report 2018 (University of Bristol Norah Fry Centre for Disability Studies, 2019) noted the median age of death for people with a learning disability (from April 2017–December 2018) was 59 years for females and 60 years for males; a disparity of 27 years for females and 23 years for males when compared to the general population. Inequities within healthcare for those with a learning disability have been raised in policies, reports and acts, yet very little progress has been made in reducing these (Department of Health, 2001; Mencap, 2007; Department of Health, 2009; The Parliamentary and Health Service Ombudsman, 2009; Mencap, 2012; Heslop et al., 2013).

More recently, providing equitable and accessible healthcare for people with a learning disability has become more prominent within allied health professions. Truly individualised and personalised care for individuals with cancer and disability has been demonstrated within therapeutic radiography departments (Johnson, 2008), yet barriers to accessing this care are still prevalent (Dodd and Dingle, 2019). The NHS long-term plan (NHS, 2019) covering the ten years from 2019 to 2029, set out methods to reduce health inequalities, including allocating Long Term Plan funding to 'ensure people with learning disability get better support'. Implementation of the 'Oliver McGowan mandatory training in learning disabilities' which has recently gained parliamentary approval and been passed into law (Health and Care Act, 2022) may help to widen understanding and awareness within allied health professions of the needs of individuals with learning disabilities and help promote true person-centred care and values-based practice for all.

Equity of access

Despite cancer, in some cases, becoming a more long-term illness which is managed across decades, cancer is still feared more than other potentially fatal diagnoses including coronary heart disease, which has approximately double the fatality rate (Alder et al., 2009). A survey of 2000 UK adults in 2010 revealed that 85% of the general public perceive that radiotherapy is inaccurate and 40% associated radiotherapy with the word 'frightening', compared to only 16% for targeted cancer drugs (Goodman, 2013). Public awareness of historic radiation incidents such as Chernobyl (1986) and Fukushima Daiichi (2011), alongside radiotherapy incidents such as the unintended overexposure of a person with cancer in Glasgow (2015), have led to negative connotations being associated with radiation, and therefore the use of radiation as a treatment. Reducing the fear and uncertainty around radiotherapy treatment is essential for all people, though additional time for preparation may be required for those with additional needs, such as learning disabilities.

Sadly, a label of a learning disability alongside outdated views of radiotherapy treatment, can result in an assumption that an individual cannot manage radiotherapy treatment, even when this is the only suitable treatment for their cancer. This has been shown in a report on LeDeR reviews involving a cancer diagnosis (Randle and Tunmore, 2018) and illustrated in a case study by Dodd and Dingle (2019). However, as shown in both this case study, and the case of a person with testicular cancer and both physical and learning disabilities detailed by Johnson (2008), adjustments to the length of appointment times, individualised care and close liaison with carers and healthcare professionals can result in individuals who are currently being deemed 'not for treatment' due to mental capacity assessments, potentially receiving curative radiotherapy. This raises the question as to whether mental capacity assessments are being conducted accurately as per the Mental Capacity Act (2005) and could mean that healthcare professionals may have to advocate for individuals to receive appropriate care which is in their best interests.

Radiotherapy treatment: understanding the basics so that you can prepare the individual with a learning disability

People with a cancer diagnosis who may benefit from radiotherapy will be referred to a clinical oncologist for assessment. Thorough clinical examination including medical history, performance status and concurrent conditions, diagnostic imaging and histological information relating to the tumour and any previous radiotherapy treatment must all be taken into consideration when deciding if radiotherapy is an appropriate treatment choice (Barrett et al., 2009). Depending on the stage and extent of the tumour, the radiotherapy treatment may be radical or palliative in intent and may be given alongside cytotoxic chemotherapy and/or pre- or post-surgical intervention (Wells, 2003). Radiotherapy works by causing damage to the DNA of cells, preventing mitosis and therefore growth of the tumour. A single, extremely high dose of radiation to a tumour would effectively destroy it; however, this would result in the death of the individual. Therefore, the dose given must be limited by the radiation tolerance doses of the surrounding organs at risk (OAR) to avoid irreparable damage to them, and therefore unmanageable side effects for the person (Munro, 2003). This must be accounted for in the planning of the treatment to achieve tumour cell kill, whilst maintaining mobility and function (and therefore quality of life) for the individual. Treating a person with cancer once daily for a number of weeks tends to promote the best response to treatment, whilst also allowing healthy cells (which proliferate more slowly) time to repair DNA damage before mitosis (Baskar et al., 2012). A radiotherapy treatment course may be delivered over varying schedules, from as little as one day to as many as eight weeks, depending on the nature of the condition and the area required for treatment.

The first stage of radiotherapy treatment is called localisation. This is where the extent of the tumour is defined using a CT scan of the area of the body where the tumour is known to be located. Contrast agents may be given to enhance the images

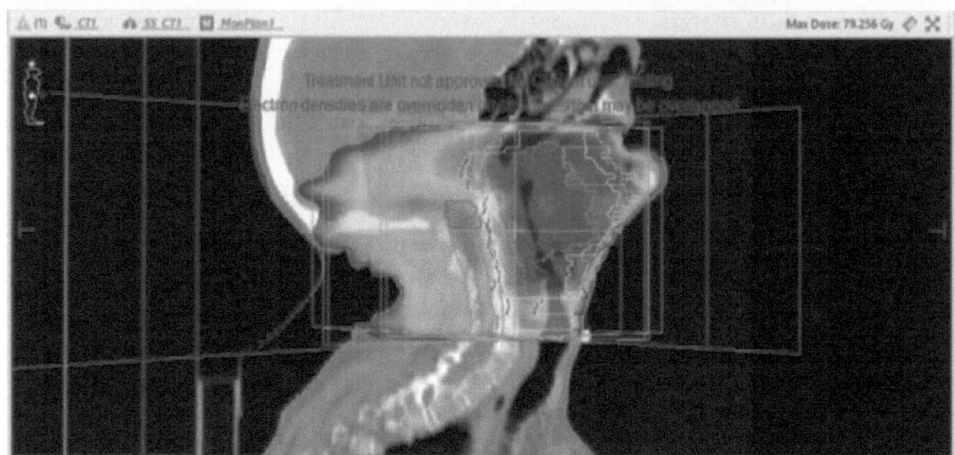

FIGURE 12.2 Head and neck radiotherapy plan (Elekta, 2023)

(Barrett et al., 2009) and, as this scan is for therapeutic not diagnostic purposes, it is conducted by therapeutic radiographers not diagnostic radiographers. This CT scan will be a simulation of the actual radiotherapy treatment, therefore the individual must be in exactly the same position for the radiotherapy treatment as for the CT localisation scan and will need to undertake any preparations required at CT for each day of radiotherapy treatment itself, such as bladder filling and deep inspiration breath hold (DIBH) techniques (see the section entitled 'Minimising side effects of radiotherapy treatment through preparation'). Once the treatment position has been determined, small tattoo dots are applied to the skin, to create a permanent reference point for future treatment set-up.

Once the CT scan is acquired, it is sent to the planning department for a process known as contouring, where a clinical oncologist will delineate the target volume, or area for treatment, on each CT slice.

The clinical oncologist will decide the radiation dose and fractionation (how many times the treatment plan will be delivered) and the plan will be checked by an independent physicist or planning therapeutic radiographer (Barrett et al., 2009). Once agreed, the plan is ready for use (see Figure 12.3).

Minimising side effects of radiotherapy treatment through preparation

Side effects from radiotherapy treatment can be caused by irradiating small areas of organs at risk (which is unavoidable when ensuring the target area is fully included in the irradiated area) and the side effect caused will be specific to the OAR. For example, irradiating some of the bowel when treating the prostate will cause diarrhoea, irradiating the skin when treating the brain will cause alopecia (in the treated area only) and irradiating the oral mucosa and salivary glands when treating the tongue will result in xerostomia and painful mucositis, often leading to oral thrush.

Side effects are cumulative as the radiation continues to kill both tumour and health cells, and so do not tend to appear in the first few weeks of treatment. If an individual is receiving a short course of radiotherapy, the side effects may not present until after their treatment is complete. Similarly, treatment side effects continue after the radiotherapy has finished, usually for up to a few weeks. Careful monitoring of the individual both during and after radiotherapy treatment is essential, especially if there are communication difficulties. Liaison with the therapeutic radiographers post-treatment and with the individual's general practitioner will be crucial to ensuring their comfort and quality of life in the final weeks of treatment and after treatment has finished. All side effects can be managed with lifestyle advice and drug therapies, but reducing the occurrence and extent of these effects in the first place is preferable.

Treatments are planned to millimetre accuracy so a small shift in a person's position can have significant consequences. Giving treatment to the incorrect area not only gives radiation dose to healthy tissues, but also reduces the dose given to the tumour, lessening the chance of achieving the desired outcome. Therefore, the drive to develop techniques to minimise organ motion and variation in the position of mobile organs has led to more complicated treatment preparation for individuals to undertake. For example, bladder-filling techniques (where the bladder is emptied, then a predetermined amount of water is consumed prior to treatment, to fill and elevate the bladder away from the prostate treatment area) have reduced radiation induced cystitis and improved people's quality of life. However, the added factor of maintaining a full bladder for up to 20 minutes while also undergoing radiotherapy treatment can cause a lot of anxiety and distress for the individual. Compliance rates vary (Smith et al., 2022), although this has improved through the use of education, especially with visual pre-treatment information delivery.

Breast cancer treatment plans can also be detrimentally impacted by organ motion through breathing during the radiotherapy delivery. Deep inspiration breath hold (DIBH) was initially developed because it was found that pausing breathing during radiation delivery meant that both heart and lung volume within the target area would be reduced (Bartlett et al., 2013). DIBH involves the individual breathing in and holding their breath during the time the radiation beam is on. However, this can be quite difficult to maintain and so practising this before radiotherapy treatment starts would reduce the stress and fear a person may feel when attempting this during their treatment.

As well as minimising internal organ motion, a variety of external immobilisation devices are used in radiotherapy treatment to prevent larger movements. These include a 'breast board' for positioning and immobilising people having their breast or chest wall irradiated, perforated thermoplastic shells for immobilising the highly moveable head and neck areas, 'vacuum bags' which can be moulded around various areas of the body to immobilise them and 'stocks' with a knee pillow to immobilise pelvic treatment areas (see Figures 12.3, 12.4, 12.5 and 12.6). Each of these devices is personalised to the individual to provide as much comfort as possible, whilst reproducing the treatment position determined at the localisation CT scan as accurately as possible (White and White, 2020). As can be seen from the images, these devices can appear quite intimidating or frightening and so familiarisation prior to radiotherapy treatment will be crucial to the individual feeling comfortable enough to undergo the procedure.

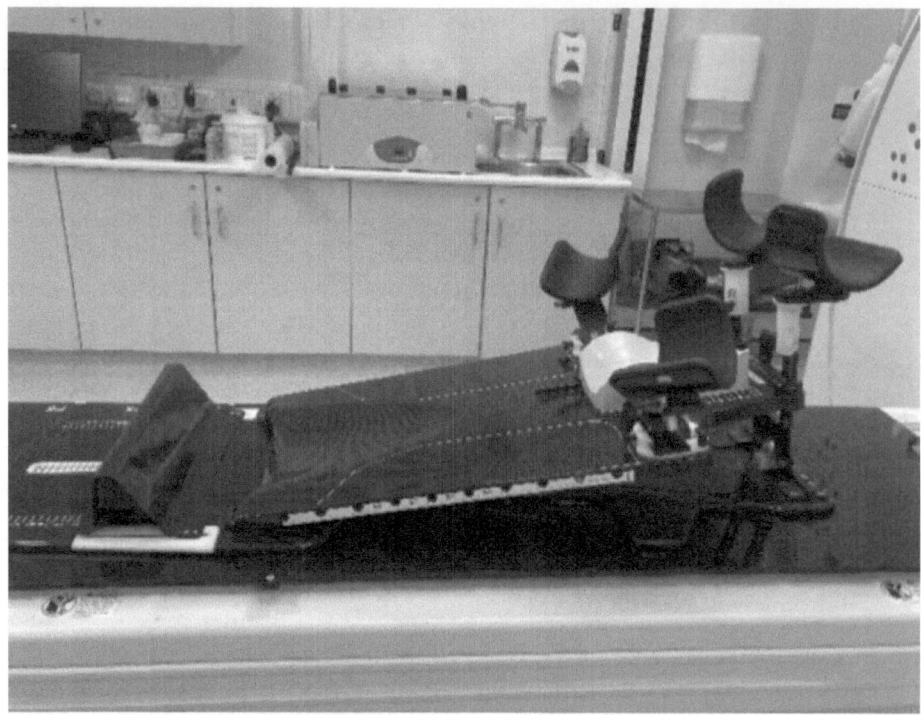

FIGURE 12.3 A radiotherapy treatment 'breast board'

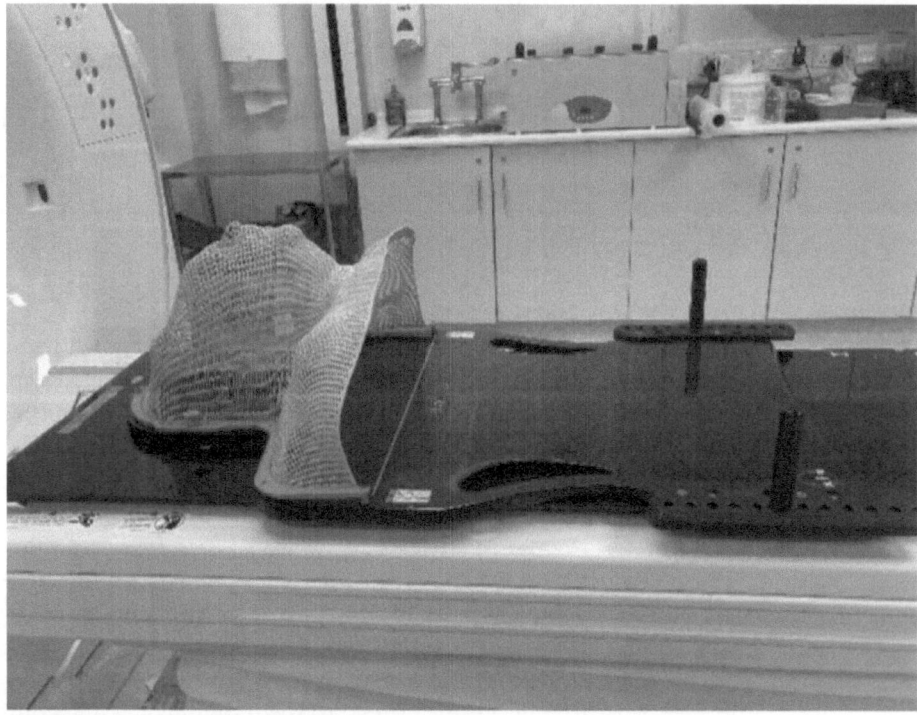

FIGURE 12.4 An 'Orfit' shell for head and neck radiotherapy

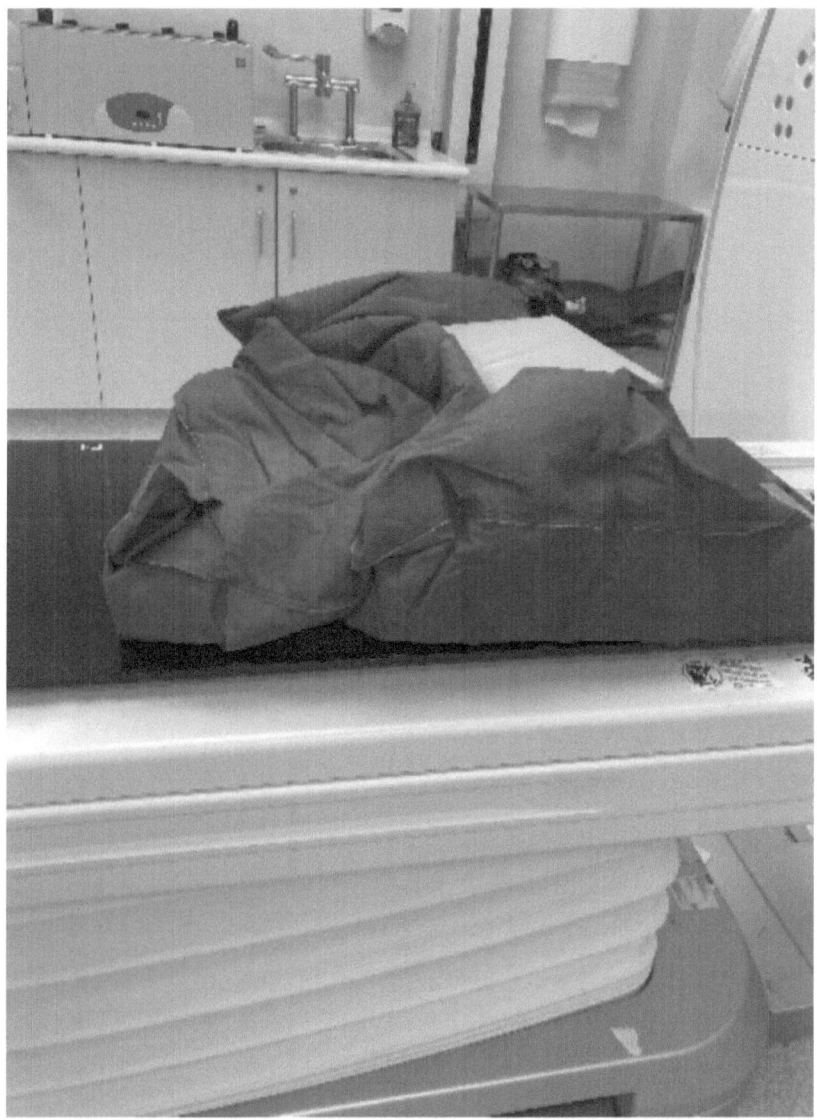

FIGURE 12.5 A vacuum bag (or 'vac bag')

Now that you have an understanding of the process – these easy read resources from Macmillan Cancer Support would be useful to help you prepare and support the individual with a learning disability: https://www.macmillan.org.uk/cancer-information-and-support/treatment/types-of-treatment/radiotherapy.

Chapter 5 by Katie Meah ('Learning from Lives and Deaths of People with Learning Disability and Autistic People – the National LeDeR Programme in Practice') gives this top tip:

It is important that you are aware of the different services that support people. When you are working with someone, it is important to know who else is

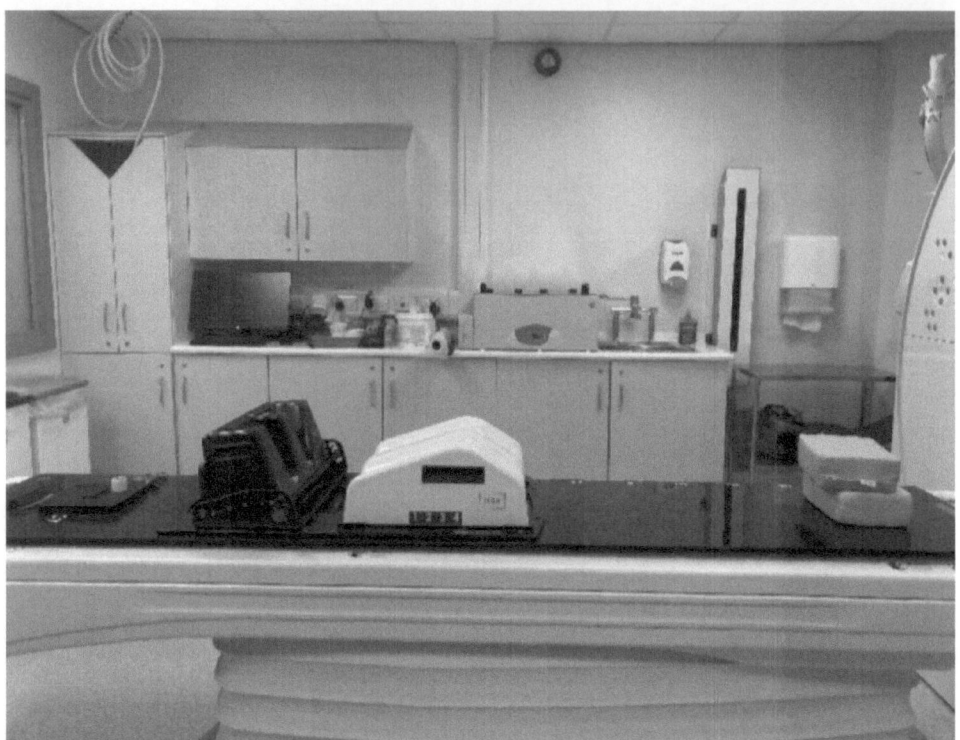

FIGURE 12.6 Foot stocks and knee pillow for pelvic treatments

involved, so that you can work together and coordinate care and ensure it is person centred.

Helping people cope with blood tests, health screening, manage their fear of needles can be achieved through desensitisation. The same thought processes can be applied to help the individual cope with maintaining the correct position.

The daily treatment process

Knowing what to expect yourselves can help you prepare the individual. Don't forget that Chapter 6 by Amanda Glennon ('Inclusive Communication: Creating Positive Outcomes – A Mother's Lived Experience') and Chapter 7 by Linda Woodcock ('Autism and Learning Disabilities') offer practical advice. This includes the importance of preparing the individual for their hospital visit, the importance of effective communication such as Makaton and top tips for communication and social interaction, using visual symbols, using schedules, providing structure and predictability, using low-arousal approaches, using hospital passports, and working with families and carers within an individualised framework of making reasonable adjustments.

Chapter 11 by Andrea Page, Alison Warren and Helen Jones ('Clinical Holding') could be referred to help you prepare the individual and gain consent and/or help you have a meaningful discussion about using clinical holding to help hold the individual still. Chapter 13 by Dr Andrew McDonnell ('Managing Distressed Behaviours in Healthcare Settings: Applying Low-Arousal Approaches') offers practical advice on dealing with distressed behaviours, which may be extremely helping when dealing with anxiety and fear of the unknown.

On each day of treatment, the individual will be called from the waiting room and taken into the treatment room. Clothing may need to be removed appropriate to the area of treatment and this may happen in a changing room outside the treatment room, or within the treatment room itself. The individual will be asked to lie on the treatment couch (bed) in the same position as they were for their localisation CT scan, having completed any pre-treatment preparation required, and using the same immobilisation devices as they were scanned with. The therapeutic radiographers move the treatment couch closer to the machine, including raising the height of the couch. They will dim the room lights and turn on laser lights, which allow them to straighten the person through the tattoo dots given at localisation, to reproduce the scan position exactly. These lasers do not provide any radiotherapy treatment themselves. The therapeutic radiographers work as a team in the treatment room, calling out instructions and measurements to each other. After checking these measurements against the treatment plan, and only once they are satisfied that all parameters are accurate, the therapeutic radiographers will inform the individual that they will be leaving the treatment room. This is in order to protect staff from repeated exposures to radiation throughout the course of each working day. The person is monitored from outside the treatment room by live cameras in the 'control area' whilst the treatment is delivered and can raise their arm or call out should they need the treatment to stop and the therapeutic radiographers to return.

Whilst the treatment is delivered, the machine will move in either a continuous arc around the person or will move to different positions in a 360-degree range of motion and then stop to deliver the treatment beam. The machine makes a quiet noise whilst it is in motion, and there is usually an artificial noise to signify that the radiation beam is on. The room lights remain dimmed with the laser lights on so that any movements made by the individual during treatment can be detected from the control area. Should this happen, the therapeutic radiographers would stop the treatment and return to the treatment room to re-set up the person. The radiation cannot be seen though there is occasionally a smell of ozone as the radiation interacts with particles in the air, especially if the radiotherapy treatment is being delivered to an area near the nose.

Particularly at the start of the treatment course, the therapeutic radiographers can take X-ray images of the treatment area, usually daily to begin with. These images are not diagnostic quality so they cannot be used to determine whether the treatment is effective or not, but they are very useful in determining treatment accuracy. Once these images are consistently showing accurate treatment they do not need to be repeated as often.

With external beam radiotherapy treatments (EBRT), the radiation dose is only present whilst the treatment beam is switched on. It is important to note that if a person has visited the nuclear medicine department, they will require the implementation of radiation protection processes, since they have ingested a 'live' radioactive source for the purpose of cancer treatment or diagnostic image acquisition. They will therefore be radioactive until the live source is excreted from their body and the remaining radiation decays to safe levels. Any waste from the individual will also be radioactive. However, with EBRT the person does not become radioactive and is safe to be around others, including children. The therapeutic radiographers will return to the treatment room, lower the treatment couch and assist the individual off the couch. The person can then get dressed and go home, unless they need to see a review therapeutic radiographer or doctor, to assess their progress through treatment and offer support and medication for any treatment side effects. The individual must return the next day and every weekday until their treatment is complete.

Supporting the individual

Careful planning and liaison between the individual (and their carers, relatives, spouse), social workers, learning disability nurse, doctors, therapeutic radiographers and other professionals involved in their care will enable optimal preparation prior to treatment, facilitating a smoother treatment journey (Randle and Tunmore, 2018) (see Table 12.1). Visiting a radiotherapy department for an out-of-hours 'walk-through' or 'dummy run' before localisation or treatment commences is the best way for everyone involved to understand what the treatment entails and can make a significant difference to how comfortable an individual will feel in such an unusual and unfamiliar environment, reducing fear of the unknown. Therapeutic radiographers can also contribute to or provide social stories and can schedule longer appointment times for quieter, less overwhelming times, such as at the start or end of the day.

Involving the person themselves is crucial to building trust and facilitating inclusion (McCann and Forbat, 2007). Should the person have a learning disability passport or other document detailing their needs, this must be brought to every appointment. Should a different means of communication be required then alerting the therapeutic radiographers in advance can enable this to happen, be this through an interpreter, or a Makaton trained signer, or provision of other communication tools such as PECS, easy-read symbols, adapted information leaflets or information provided in visual formats.

Adaptations can also be made to the localisation, immobilisation and treatment process to aid comfort and manageability. For example, alternative ways of immobilising the person can be considered, the requirement for treatment preparation such as bladder filling can be removed and shorter treatment regimes can be implemented. Familiar music can be played and comforting scents can be introduced to the treatment room and home items can be brought, such as a blanket to cover areas not being treated. Sometimes a reassuring object can either be held or placed in close proximity. Any reasonable adjustment that does not significantly compromise the treatment should be implemented.

TABLE 12.1 Questions to ask pre-radiotherapy treatment

Questions for learning disability nurses to ask	Questions for therapeutic radiographers to ask
Has a mental capacity assessment been undertaken appropriately?	Can the person manage the requirements of the standard care pathway or treatment protocol?
What pre-treatment requirements does the person need to achieve?	Can a pre-localisation and pre-treatment visit be arranged for the individual?
Can a visit be arranged to the department so that the treatment process can be seen and understood by the person's carers, so that explanation and preparation for treatment can take place?	What is the best method of communication for the person? Is written information required in a specific format?
Can continuity of accompanying staff be achieved?	Does the person have a 'My Care Passport' with them?
Is there a point of contact for pre-attendance discussions, to ensure a smooth treatment experience?	What would constitute the best environment possible in which the person would receive their treatment (quieter, calmer, longer appointment times, at a department close to home, etc.)?
Is the person's hospital passport/My Care Passport available to take to the radiotherapy department daily?	Can continuity of people (both staff within the radiotherapy department and carers) be achieved?
Is liaison required to ensure optimal communication?	Can a named individual co-ordinate the care of the person?
Does a social story need preparing in conjunction with the therapeutic radiographers?	Is it possible to achieve a consistent routine within the radiotherapy department, treatment room and for appointment times?
What 'home items', music, scents, etc. could be brought to the treatment room to ensure the person feels as comfortable as possible?	What else could be suggested or recommended to ensure the person feels as comfortable as possible?

The introduction of a learning disability therapeutic radiography lead role would be a welcome addition to the specialisms available to therapeutic radiographers, and would enable much smoother coordination of care pathways for people with a learning disability. A therapeutic radiographer in this role would be able to ensure appropriate training for all staff members, liaise with other healthcare professionals involved in the individual's care and manage effective day-to-day radiotherapy treatment of people with a learning disability.

Equitable and accessible care is a basic right for all individuals. Flexibility and adaptability are key to ensuring inclusive and appropriate care can be delivered to all people, even if this means that the 'optimal' radiotherapy treatment procedure cannot be achieved. Delivering the best possible care, given in the person's best interests *is* the optimal treatment, and working outside of standard protocol may be essential.

Resources

Birmingham City University's Clinical Holding Guide. Available at: https://chg. osimebcu.co.uk

Cornwall Down's Syndrome Support Group (CDSSG) *Going to Hospital* book. Available at: Going to Hospital Book - Cornwall Down's Syndrome Support Group (cdssg.org.uk)

NHS Accessible Information Standard. Available at: https://www.england.nhs.uk/ about/equality/equality-hub/patient-equalities-programme/equality-frame-works-and-information-standards/accessibleinfo/

Macmillan Cancer Support would be useful to help you prepare and support the individual with a learning disability. Available at: https://www.macmillan.org. uk/cancer-information-and-support/treatment/types-of-treatment/radiotherapy

References

Alder, B., Abraham, C., van Teijlingen, E. and Porter, M. (2009) *Psychology and Sociology Applied to Medicine*, 3rd edition. Edinburgh: Churchill Livingstone Elsevier. Available at: https:// r1.vlereader.com/Reader?ean=9780702048203 [Accessed 17 January 2024].

Barrett, A., Dobbs, J., Morris, S. and Roques, T. (2009) *Practical Radiotherapy Planning*, 4th edition. London: Hodder Arnold.

Bartlett, F.R., Colgan, R.M., Carr, K., Donovan, E.M., McNair, H.A., Locke, I., Evans, P.M., Haviland, J.S., Yarnold, J.R. and Kirby, A.M. (2013) The UK HeartSpare Study: Randomised evaluation of voluntary deep-inspiratory breath-hold in women undergoing breast radiotherapy. *Radiotherapy and Oncology*, 108(2). Available at: https://www.science direct.com/science/article/pii/S0167814013001965 [Accessed 14 February 2024].

Baskar, R., Lee, K.A., Yoe, R. and Yoeh, K.-W. (2012) Cancer and radiation therapy: Current advances and future directions. *International Journal of Medical Sciences*, 9(3). Available at: https://www.ncbi.nlm.nih.gov/pmc/articles/PMC3298009/ [Accessed 17 January 2024].

Department of Health (2001) *Valuing People: A New Strategy for Learning Disability for the 21st Century*. [pdf] Available at: https://assets.publishing.service.gov.uk/government/uploads/ system/uploads/attachment_data/file/250877/5086.pdf [Accessed 5 January 2023].

Department of Health (2009) *Valuing People Now: Summary Report March 2009–September 2010*. [pdf] Available at: https://assets.publishing.service.gov.uk/government/uploads/system/ uploads/attachment_data/file/215891/dh_122387.pdf [Accessed 5 January 2023].

Dodd, A. and Dingle, E. (2019) Case Study – Supporting a man with learning difficulties to receive radiotherapy. *Radiography*, 26(1). Available at: https://www.radiographyonline. com/article/S1078-8174(19)30176-2/fulltext [Accessed 5 January 2023].

Duffton, A., Li, W. and Forde, E. (2020) The pivotal role of the therapeutic radiographer/ radiation therapist in image-guided radiotherapy research and development. *Clinical Oncology*, 32(12). Available at https://www.sciencedirect.com/science/article/pii/S093665552 0303708 [Accessed 17 January 2024].

Elekta (2023) Monaco Training System, Stockholm. https://www.elekta.com/

Goodman, S. (2013) A guide to modern radiotherapy. Available at: https://www.sor.org/learning/ document-library/guide-modern-radiotherpy [Accessed 17 January 2024].

Health and Care Act 2022, part 6: 181 Available at: https://www.legislation.gov.uk/ukpga/2022/31/contents/enacted [Accessed 17 January 2024].

Heslop. P., Blair, P., Fleming, P., Hoghton, M., Marriott, A. and Russ, L. (2013) *The Confidential Inquiry into Premature Deaths of People with Learning Disabilities.* [pdf] Available at: http://www.bris.ac.uk/media-library/sites/cipold/migrated/documents/fullfinalreport.pdf [Accessed 17 January 2024].

Holt, A (2017) Disabled man's cancer care criticised. BBC News, 15 December. Available at: https://www.bbc.co.uk/news/health-42339856 [Accessed 5 January 2024].

Johnson, J. (2008) A case of...seminoma in a patient with disabilities. *Synergy: Imaging and Therapy Practice.* [pdf] June, 8–11 [archived].

McCann, L and Forbat, L (2007) *Older People with Learning Disabilities Affected by Cancer: Involvement and Engagement Work to Inform a Research Agenda.* [pdf] Available at: https://dspace.stir.ac.uk/bitstream/1893/12739/1/Forbat_2007_Older_people_with_learning_disabilities_affected_by_cancer.pdf [Accessed 9 February 2024].

Mencap (2007) *Death by Indifference.* [pdf] Available at: https://www.mencap.org.uk/sites/default/files/2016-07/DBIreport.pdf [Accessed 17 January 2024].

Mencap (2012) *Death by Indifference: 74 Deaths and Counting.* [pdf] Available at: https://www.mencap.org.uk/sites/default/files/2016-08/Death%20by%20Indifference%20-%2074%20deaths%20and%20counting.pdf [Accessed 17 January 2024].

Mental Capacity Act 2005, Part 1. Available at: https://www.legislation.gov.uk/ukpga/2005/9/contents [Accessed 14 February 2024].

Munro, A.J. (2003) Challenges to radiotherapy today. In S. Faithfull and M. Wells (eds) *Supportive Care in Radiotherapy.* Edinburgh: Churchill Livingstone, pp. 17–38.

NHS (2019) *The NHS Long Term Plan.* Available at: https://www.longtermplan.nhs.uk/online-version/overview-and-summary/ [Accessed 9 February 2023].

Parliamentary and Health Service Ombudsman (2009) *Six Lives: The Provision of Public Services to People with Learning Difficulties 2008 to 2009.* [pdf] Available at: https://assets.publishing.service.gov.uk/government/uploads/system/uploads/attachment_data/file/250750/0203.pdf [Accessed 17 January 2024].

Patja, K., Eero, P. and Iivanainen, M. (2001) Cancer incidence among people with intellectual disability. *Journal of Intellectual Disability Research*, 45(4). Available at: https://doi-org.bcu.idm.oclc.org/10.1046/j.1365-2788.2001.00322 [Accessed 9 January 2024].

Randle, A. and Tunmore, R. (2018) *Learning into Action – Report on LeDeR Reviews Involving a Cancer Diagnosis.* [pdf] Available at https://northerncanceralliance.nhs.uk/wp-content/uploads/2020/08/LearningIntoActionReport.pdf [Accessed 14 February 2024].

Smith, L., Gittins, J., Ramnarine, K.V. and Chung, E.M.L. (2022) Assessment of an ultrasound bladder scanner in prostate radiotherapy: A validation study and analysis of bladder filling variability. *Ultrasound.* 30(1). Available at: https://www.ncbi.nlm.nih.gov/pmc/articles/PMC8841937/ [Accessed 14 February 2024].

Spencer, K., Hole, D., Symonds, P. and Morris, E. (2019) Epidemiology of cancer and screening. In P. Symonds, J.A. Mills and A. Duxbury (eds) *Walter and Millers Textbook of Radiotherapy: Radiation Physics, Therapy and Oncology.* 8th edition. Edinburgh: Churchill Livingstone, pp. 226–238.

Sullivan, S.G., Hussain, R., Threlfall, T. and Bittles, A.H. (2004) The incidence of cancer in people with intellectual disabilities. *Cancer Causes & Control*, 15(10). Available at: https://www-jstor-org.bcu.idm.oclc.org/stable/pdf/3553584 [Accessed 9 February 2024].

Symonds, P., Deehan, C., Meredith, C. and Mills, J. (2012) *Walter and Miller's Textbook of Radiotherapy: Radiation Physics, Therapy and Oncology.* 7th edition. Edinburgh: Elsevier Churchill Livingstone.

Tuffrey-Wijne, I. (2010) *Living with Learning Disabilities, Dying with Cancer : Thirteen Personal Stories.* London: Jessica Kingsley

University of Bristol Norah Fry Centre for Disability Studies (2019) *The Learning Disability Mortality Review (LeDeR) Programme Annual Report 2018*. [pdf] Available at: https://www. bristol.ac.uk/media-library/sites/sps/leder/LeDeR_Annual_Report_2018%20pub lished%20May%202019.pdf [Accessed 17 January 2024].

Wells, M. (2003) The treatment trajectory. In S. Faithfull and M. Wells (eds) *Supportive Care in Radiotherapy*. Edinburgh: Churchill Livingstone, pp. 39–59.

White, H.P. and White, N. (2020) Principles of treatment accuracy and reproducibility. In P. Cherry and A.M. Duxbury (eds) *Practical Radiotherapy: Physics and Equipment*. Chichester: John Wiley and Sons, pp. 111–143.

Wood, A. (2018) People with learning disabilities face gross inequity in life and death. *The Guardian*, 29 May. Available at: https://www.theguardian.com/social-care-network/2018/may/29/learning-disabilities-inequality-life-death-leder-report [Accessed 5 January 2024].

13

Managing distressed behaviours in healthcare settings

Applying Low Arousal Approaches

Andrew McDonnell

Managing distressed behaviours in healthcare settings: applying Low Arousal Approaches

In their lifetime, many people in society will experience distressed behaviour, which can often take the form of verbal and physical aggression. In healthcare settings, healthcare workers, including nurses, are often expected to support distressed individuals on a daily basis. Healthcare settings in the UK can be highly stressful environments, ranging from GP surgeries to Accident and Emergency departments. Managing distressed behaviours in a calm and regulated manner is an essential skill for frontline nurses and other healthcare practitioners. For nurses supporting people with a learning disability or autism, the challenge is to manage stressful situations in a dignified and empathic manner. Many of the people who require our support have often experienced significant trauma and distress in their lives (McDonnell, 2019). Supporting individuals who are vulnerable is a significant challenge. This chapter will discuss some of the common misconceptions about and causes of distressed behaviour, as well as describe and apply a collection of support strategies known as Low Arousal Approaches to managing distressed behaviours. This will include practical tips for applying the Low Arousal Approach in healthcare settings when individuals become distressed, and strategies to use within hospital settings.

Distressed Behaviour and Crisis Situations

Learning disability nurses in their day-to-day practice often support individuals who are distressed and experiencing 'meltdown' (Lipsky, 2011) and have therefore been seen as specialists in behaviour management. Following the changes to nursing education all fields of nursing upon qualifying are expected to demonstrate

DOI: 10.4324/9781003341765-15

proficiency in assessing, delivering and evaluating care of individuals experiencing 'mental and emotional distress including agitation, aggression and challenging behaviour' (NMC, 2018). In most circumstances, the distress that people experience is not always targeted towards the nurse or other practitioners, and can be due to a range of factors, including: pain, deterioration in physical health, physical discomfort (compounded by interoceptive difficulties), environmental stressors and emotional distress. Managing these meltdowns requires individuals to create a non-threatening environment. Sometimes crisis situations are influenced by the clinical environment, meaning that nurses are expected to create a calm environment to provide treatment or interventions to distressed individuals. These can range from talking to people, to having to clinically hold an individual (Page et al., 2019).

Student nurses in training can be exposed to many distressing behaviours and situations, sometimes even from their own peers. Research in the UK has shown that incivility (here defined as rude, disruptive or undesirable behaviours) in classroom and clinical settings disrupts learning, as well as impacting on student nurse wellbeing and patient outcomes (Vuolo, 2017). This is almost certainly an international problem. A study conducted in Hong Kong found that, of 1017 nursing students surveyed, 37.3% reported having experienced clinical violence during their nursing studies (Cheung, Ching, Cheng & Ho, 2019). The prevalence of verbal abuse was found to be significantly greater than that of physical violence. The perpetrators of verbal abuse were predominantly patients, but also included hospital staff, university supervisors and patients' relatives.

There has been a recent emphasis, especially in the National Health Service (NHS), that violence and aggression should not be tolerated in healthcare settings, which has led to an increasing number of zero tolerance policies. If you enter any NHS hospital environment, you will be confronted by warning signs and posters stating that violence and aggression towards staff will not be tolerated. The reality is that many of these policies could at best be described as ineffective. A recent study in Australia found that despite organisations having policies supporting zero tolerance, many staff do not enact these because they prioritise duty of care to consumers before duty of care to self (Beattie, Innes, Griffiths & Morphet, 2020). Zero tolerance, alongside incongruent legislation, compounds this tension and impairs decision-making.

There is also evidence that the stresses on healthcare systems created by the Covid-19 pandemic have had an impact on instances of violence and aggression. Four global health organisations, including the International Council of Nurses (ICN), surveyed their members in 2021 and found that almost 60% reported an increase in recorded instances of violence against their workforce during the pandemic (ICN et al., 2022). Stress and violence are correlated, although there is considerable debate about whether there is a causal link (Anderson & Bushman, 2002). The expression of anger and how to manage it is another common issue. In many situations, nurses are expected to deal with angry individuals. A study on anger in emergency departments found that a range of patients' anger expressions were correlated with staff fear (Arik, Anat & Arie, 2012). Staff's responses to anger from others ranged from ignoring incidents, giving in to patients' requests, or immediately calling security. Interestingly, staff whose fear led to their own feelings of anger tended to call security. Understanding and dealing with everyday anger, both in ourselves and others, is a cornerstone of good crisis management.

Dealing with our own distress

Nurses are often confronted by individuals who will be distressed. In a Swedish study, it was found that nurses who had been physically assaulted by the people they supported reported feelings of anger towards that person after the event (Lundström, Aström & Graneheim, 2007):

> The main findings indicate that caregivers' experiences of being exposed to violence can be related to two themes: falling apart, and keeping it together. Falling apart includes feelings of fear, powerlessness, sadness, anger and timelessness, while keeping it together concerns pleasure, respect, self-reflection and habituation.

Whilst many individuals who are distressed do not overtly display anger responses, in practice significant numbers of healthcare workers will be expected to manage crisis situations where distressed behaviour that is directed towards them presents as anger. Anger is a complex emotional state that can have both positive and negative elements. At some point in our lives, we will all experience angry thoughts and feelings.

AN EVERYDAY ANGER EXERCISE

The following exercise is designed to help the reader reflect on their own anger responses.
Think about the last time you were openly angry with a friend, colleague, relative, or complete stranger.
Consider the following questions:

1. On reflection, why were you angry?
2. How did your anger get resolved?
   a. Did you talk about it with the individual you were angry at?
   b. Did you just ignore the issue and move on?
   c. Is your anger unresolved?
3. Would you describe yourself as an angry person?
4. Do you think the experience of anger is acceptable in certain contexts and not others?

The above exercise is important if we are to take a reflective approach, not just of the anger that we experience from patients, but understanding our own anger first (McDonnell, 2019). Even when we analyse our own behaviour, we may not always be completely aware of other environmental factors that have had an impact. Social contexts have a huge impact on how we think and behave. Environmental factors such as crowding, noise, hostility from other individuals and group factors can all lead to angry responses. There are also many internal factors, such as our own physical health and wellbeing, which may cause us to express anger. A recent study found that everyday levels of hunger are associated with negative emotions. Results indicated that greater levels of self-reported hunger were associated with greater feelings of anger and irritability, thus supporting the notion of being 'hangry' (Swami, Hochstöger, Kargl & Stieger, 2022). It is important to understand our own anger and emotional responses, as this will contribute to how we respond to people who are hostile and distressed. In order to manage the anger of others, we must first be aware of our own triggers which may cause us to respond to or exacerbate distressing situations.

Dealing with other people's distress

There is little doubt that healthcare professionals require an understanding of how to manage and respond to distressed individuals, particularly in hospital settings where treatment is a priority. For example, in GP surgeries, distressed behaviour may be easier to manage than in an Accident and Emergency department, where treatment is more urgent and patients more frightened and scared. Nurses often develop working relationships with individuals, but there are many circumstances where they will be asked to work with complete strangers. The relationship we have with the individual is always important.

Regardless of the situation, crisis management skills should be viewed as being useful in good and bad times. Throughout their career, nurses will be expected to engage with individuals who are scared, confused, distressed and often traumatised. Having empathy for the individual you are supporting and understanding why they are distressed or appear angry is key. It is important to recognise that in crisis situations, a distressed person's emotions can become contagious (Elvén, 2010).

The impact of distressing behaviours and situations on our own emotional regulation is an area that we can, to a certain degree, control. If we can remember that people are often stressed and traumatised, it will create a sense of empathy and compassion, and have an impact on our responses. Our emotions are challenged when we experience distressed behaviour. In these circumstances, it is essential that people learn to separate their own feelings and emotions from those of the people they support. Understanding and compartmentalising these emotional reactions can help individuals to respond in a calm and regulated manner. Building trusting relationships is an essential skill for learning disability nurses, who often support individuals over their lifespan and innately take a holistic approach; supporting family and significant others as well as the person. With the aforementioned changes to nurse education there is the expectation that all nurses will be able to support a range of people with complex conditions in a variety of settings. Depending on the environment a nurse works in, this essential skill will apply to all four fields of nursing in varying degrees. The psychologist Lori Desautels has argued that people who make positive emotional connections with even the most challenging people tend to focus less on rules and compliances (Desautels, 2020). Developing trauma-informed and empathic responses to distressing situations often requires us to reflect on our own behaviour. The Low Arousal Approach to crisis management focuses on how to manage situations in the moment, and this means being aware of how we react to and learn from distressing situations. *The Reflective Journey: A Practitioner's Guide to the Low Arousal Approach* (McDonnell, 2019) states that the key to the approach is reflecting on our experiences and developing an empathic and compassionate approach to individuals who are distressed. Healthcare professionals often need to see the trauma and see the person. A simple rule is to ask yourself the question, 'How would I like to be treated in this situation?' There are other factors which are important in regulating our responses, including understanding how our autonomic nervous system links to our own physiological arousal.

Arousal regulation

It is self-evident that stressful situations where arousal levels are high can have an impact on our responses, whether we are supporting someone on their own or in group situations. During heightened states of arousal (also known as hyperarousal), the human brain can become easily overwhelmed. Porges (2011) describes the process by which our bodies respond to threats using the nervous system through polyvagal theory. Polyvagal theory refers to the process by which the autonomic nervous system uses nerve fibres to transmit information from the body toward the brain (afferent influences), and from the brain to the body (efferent influences). In many ways, individuals are victims of their own autonomic nervous system, which unconsciously influences their decision making. Polyvagal theory suggests that many of our immediate crisis responses are linked to basic survival instincts. Understanding these systems helps to create more meaningful perspectives about why people behave in the way they do. The psychologist Mona Delahooke has argued that brain science can help to explain why people sometimes behave in ways that seem almost impossible to understand (Delahooke, 2019).

Understanding the arousal mechanisms in our own bodies can help us learn to self-regulate. Porges (2011) talks about three responses to heightened states of physiological arousal, which he labels as social engagement, defensive reactions (fight or flight), or a 'life-threat' (which we would commonly call a shutdown). In this model, people are trying to adapt to the perceived stressful environment around them. In order to manage or regulate the arousal levels of distressed people, coregulation is necessary. This means that, when a person is experiencing arousal dysregulation, we need to respond in a calm and regulated manner, thus encouraging them to begin the process of calming down. Co-regulation is at the centre of the Low Arousal Approach, which at its core means role modelling calmness in order to take control of crisis situations.

Definition of the Low Arousal Approach

The Low Arousal Approach is a collection of non-aversive behaviour management strategies which focus on reducing physiological arousal as well as internal and external environmental stressors in order to avoid or de-escalate crisis situations

(McDonnell, McEvoy & Dearden, 1994; Elvén, 2010; Woodcock & Page, 2010; McDonnell, 2019, 2022). Essentially, applying a Low Arousal Approach means that supporters focus on what they can do to reduce their own physiological arousal, help regulate the arousal of others, and identify stress, trauma and other triggers that could be contributing to challenging or distressed behaviour.

McDonnell, McCreadie and Dickinson identified four key elements of the Low Arousal Approach (2019: 458–459):

> First, decreasing staff demands and requests, to reduce potential points of conflict around an individual. Second, avoidance of potentially arousing triggers (e.g., direct eye contact, and touch and removal of spectators to the incident). Third, the avoidance of non-verbal behaviours that may lead to conflict (e.g., aggressive postures and stances). Fourth, challenging staff/carer beliefs about short-term management of behaviours of concern.

The approach relies on practitioners reflecting on incidents and identifying areas where their own behaviour may have contributed to an incident. This means encouraging supporters to focus on their own stress management and arousal regulation. The aim is to create a system of support that fosters a calm and regulated environment; after all, how can we help someone to calm down when we ourselves are highly stressed? Whilst it is distressing to witness individuals in highly charged emotional incidents and not intervene, taking a moment to collect yourself and take a step back can make a huge difference to the situation. Low Arousal does not mean 'no arousal' whatsoever, but it does mean looking at these incidents in a different way. Once a calm situation has been restored, there is an opportunity for all participants to reflect and learn from the incident.

Practical Low Arousal application

There are many useful things to consider when managing a distressed person or situation. Student nurses and other healthcare professionals can reduce their perceived threat to distressed individuals by following relatively simple advice (McDonnell, 2019). The following should be seen as a guide to how to apply Low Arousal Approaches to an individual who may be in a state of extreme hyper-arousal.

Ten non-verbal Low Arousal strategies

1) Stay (or appear) calm

One important skill that a person must learn is to appear calm to people who are distressed. Just as distressed emotions and related behaviours can directly trigger similar emotions and behaviours in other people, so too can calmness be greatly influential in crisis situations. Staying calm in these situations is a skill that can be practised. The more often we respond in a calm manner, the more confident we will appear, and the safer the distressed individual will feel in our care.

2) Avoid direct eye contact

Direct eye contact can be extremely arousing, especially to people who are already distressed. It can indicate conflict, assert dominance and ultimately communicate aggression. Particularly for autistic people, direct eye contact can be difficult to process alongside other sensory stimuli such as verbal communication and background

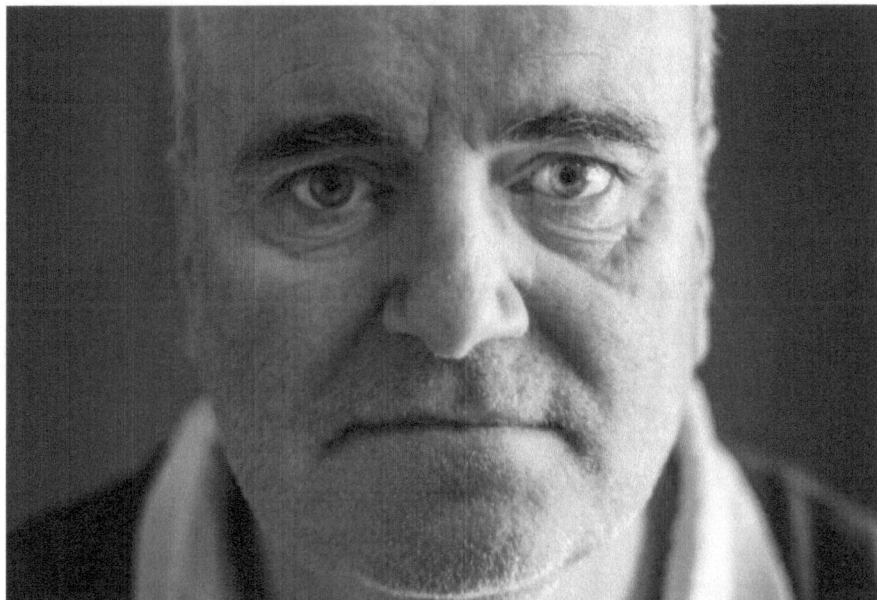

FIGURE 13.1 Eye contact

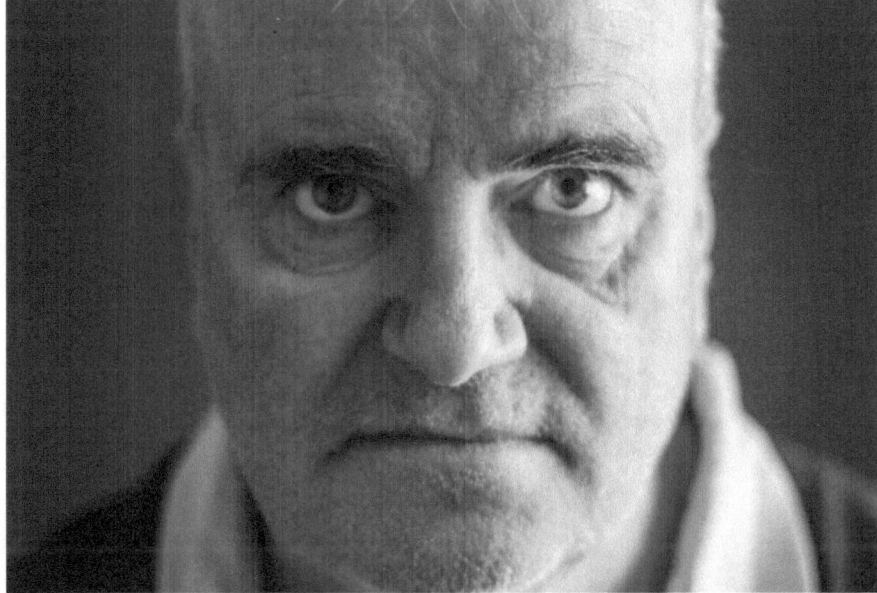

FIGURE 13.2 Direct eye contact

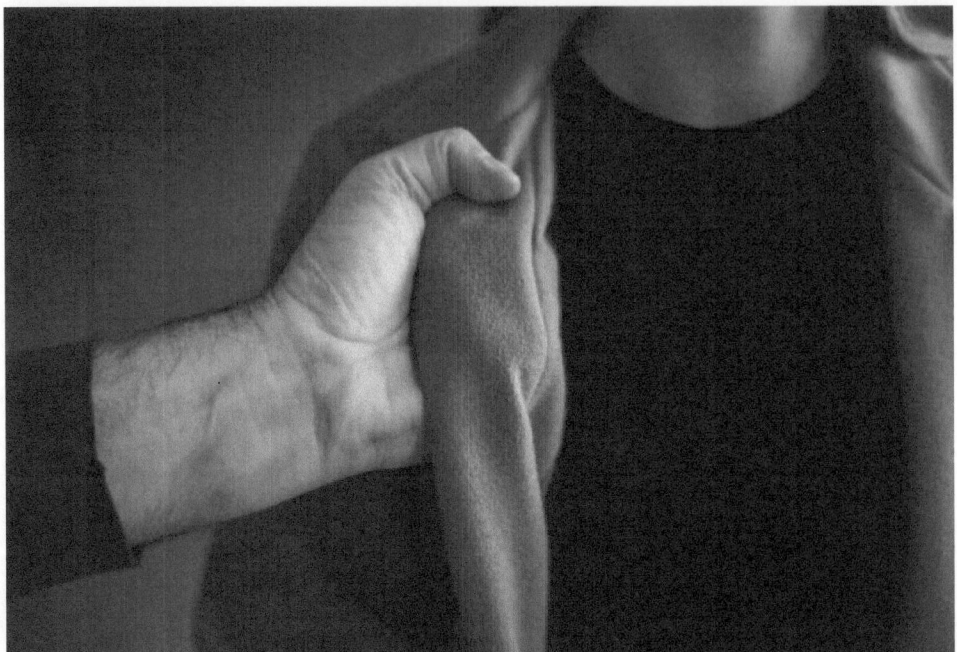

FIGURE 13.3 Physical touch

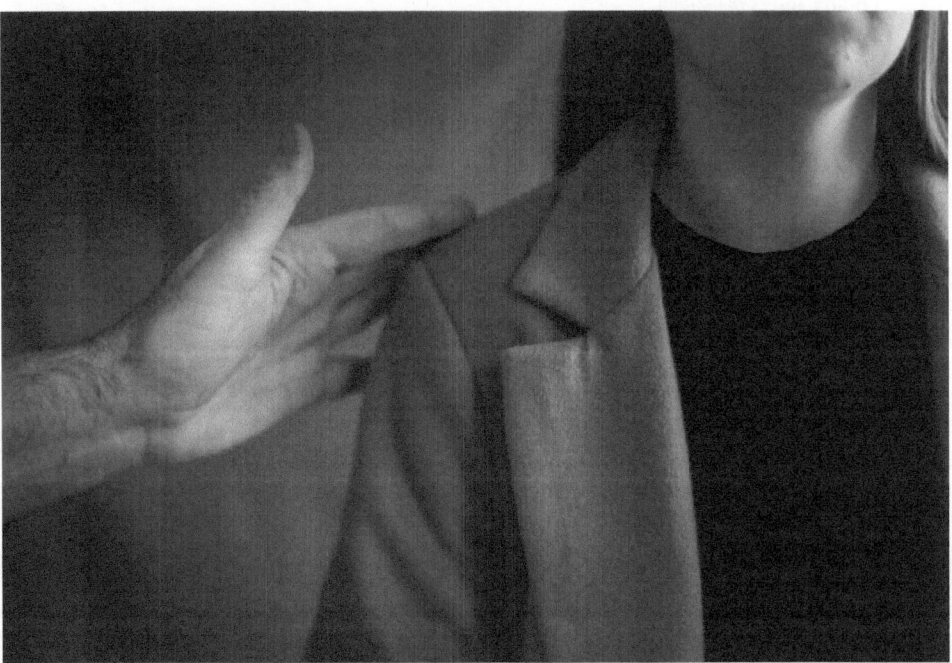

FIGURE 13.4 Shoulder touch

noises, leading to them become overwhelmed. When you are in a situation where someone is highly aroused or in 'meltdown', try to avoid staring and instead maintain regular, intermittent eye contact.

The first image depicts direct eye contact, and comes across as threatening and aggressive. The second image shows the same subject looking slightly downward, and conveys a much less threatening, passive expression.

3) Be wary of physical touch

Touch can be a sign of affection, warmth and security, but it also can be a sign of threat and hostility. When someone is highly aroused, even well-intended touch can be received as an aversive stimulus. Be mindful that individuals may have been traumatised by hospital settings in their past, or experienced restraint from a medical professional. A key part of the Low Arousal Approach is the avoidance of physical restraint, which also means the removal of the threat of restraint from the distressed person's environment.

The above images demonstrate how differently touch can be perceived when someone feels threatened.

4) Slow your movements down

Move slowly and cautiously around someone who is clearly threatened and distressed. People in a hyper-aroused state will interpret movements towards them as a threat. Let the person know in advance what you are going to do and approach them in a calm and slow manner. Appearing calm and confident here will also help.

5) Gestures can be misinterpreted

Gestures and postures are a natural part of human communication that enhance what we are expressing. Consider the images in Figures 13.5 and 13.6 and what you think they communicate. The images are examples of open and closed postures. These will often be the first signals a distressed person processes, as spoken language can be processed more slowly when a person is highly aroused. Ensuring that your posture and gestures are non-threatening, confident and calm will signal to the individual that you are not a threat.

6) Avoid gathering staff in a crisis

It is common in healthcare settings that staff will congregate in numbers when a person is showing signs of distress. 'Safety in numbers' may make staff feel safer, but it can be arousing and threatening for the distressed person. Only one person should communicate with the person, and if a second member of staff is necessary, they should be out of the individual's line of sight, and only assist if requested to do so by the lead person.

7) Remove onlookers

Traditional approaches focus on removing the distressed person from the environment, often by verbal demand or using physical restraint. It is better to avoid the 'audience effect' of being watched by others in a stressful situation (Strauss, 2002). This is more likely to escalate the situation into crisis, and may result in unnecessary

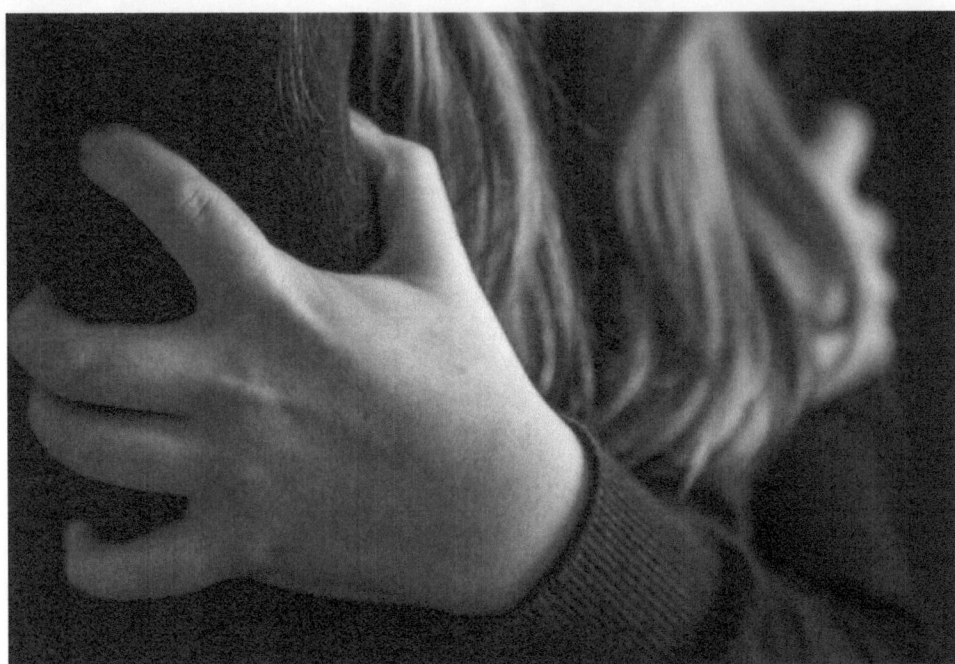

FIGURE 13.5 Arm clutch

and in some cases dangerous or unlawful physical restraint. It is, however, preferable to encourage other people to vacate the environment and to have positive and proactive strategies in place to achieve this. Removing onlookers can be the easier option, enabling the distressed person to calm down in their own time. Remember that onlookers can also be traumatised by witnessing distressing situations.

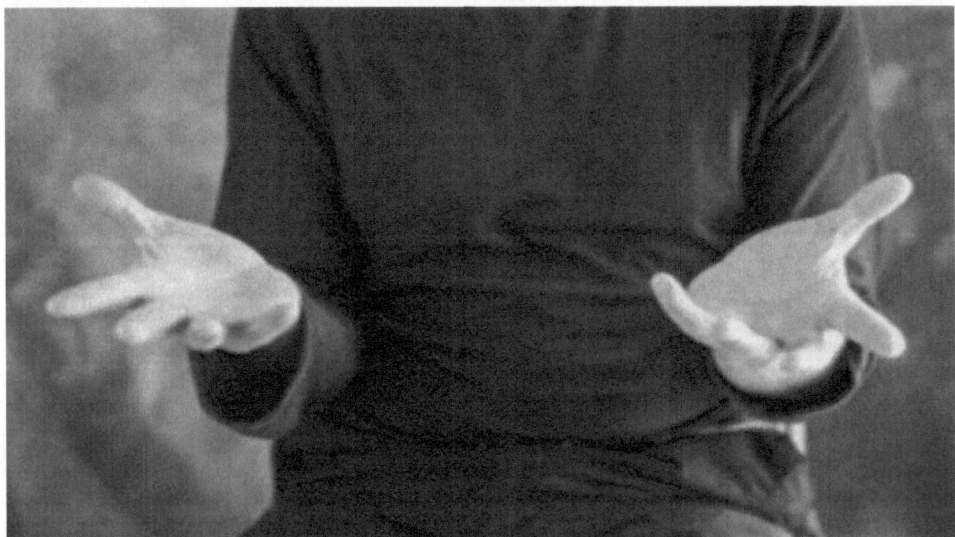

FIGURE 13.6 Open hands

8) Keep your distance

People who are highly stressed and hypervigilant are more likely to require more interpersonal space. When supporting a distressed person keep, at the very least, an arm's length away. Arousal is mostly subconscious, and someone invading your personal space will fuel the 'fight or flight' response. Polyvagal theory (Porges, 2011) suggests that people will become hyper-sensitive to even subtle invasions of their interpersonal space.

9) Be aware of the power messages you communicate

Frightened and stressed individuals are often expected to meet nurses in clinics and other healthcare settings which may evoke strong emotions of fear and distress. It is important that nurses and other healthcare professionals understand that people may be hypervigilant in these situations, and be reluctant to accept help. It is important to acknowledge that healthcare professionals do have considerable power, and patients may have negative associations with hospital and other healthcare settings in general. Try to avoid taking control in these situations, and avoid verbal and non-verbal communication that may lead to conflict and misunderstanding. Be aware of the emotion and tone and of your voice – speak slowly, calmly and softly. Keep your language simple and clear, and supplement with visual information if appropriate.

When working with young children, it is important to remember that, like in the book *Gulliver's Travels* (Swift, 1726/2003), we may appear almost as giants, and unintentionally convey threatening messages.

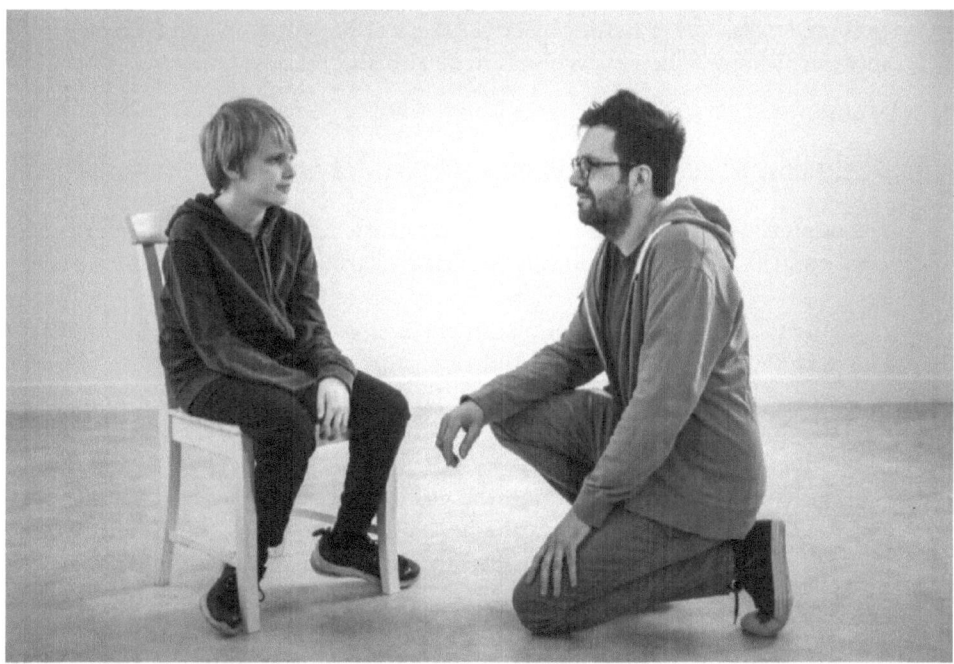

FIGURE 13.7 Boy Man eye level

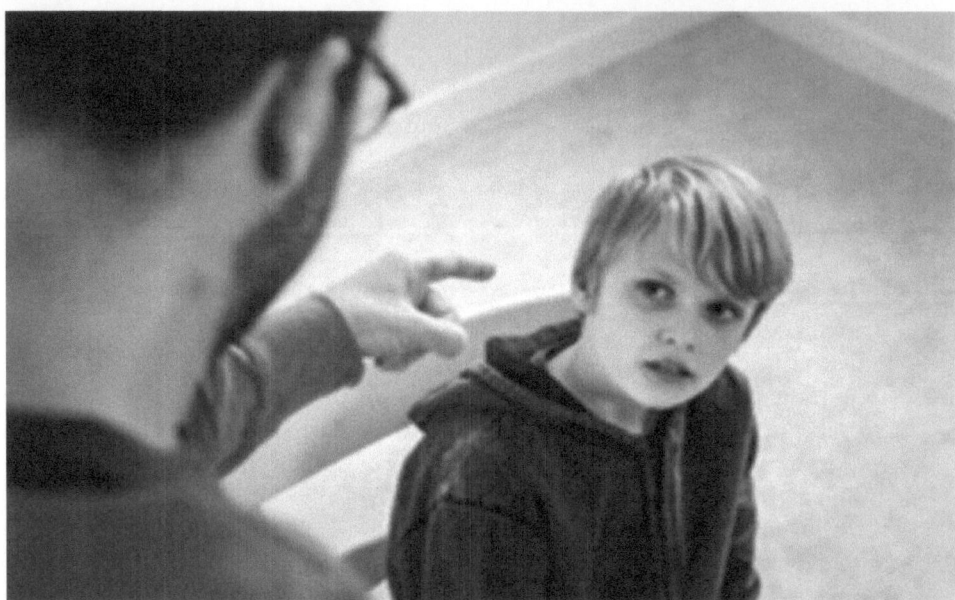

FIGURE 13.8 Man pointing at boy

10) Tactical withdrawal

Sometimes withdrawing from a situation can lead to a decrease in physiological arousal. Avoid getting involved in arguments, disputes or 'stand-offs' when someone is highly aroused. Somebody needs to back down and, more often than not, that will need to be you. Try not to view this as 'giving in' – avoiding distress and a potential crisis is the main objective. Reflection, support and learning will be far more achievable when everyone is in a calm and relaxed state.

Applying Low Arousal Approaches in hospital and healthcare settings

Encountering distressed people requires a reflective approach. Understanding our own contribution to situations is essential. Consider the following example:

Jane is a student nurse on placement in a community team, supporting people with intellectual disabilities and/or autism. As part of her studies, she attends an outreach clinic on a weekly basis. Jane was asked to gather health information about a young man with labels including complex trauma and intellectual disabilities. The young man arrived at the clinic in an agitated state. He found it difficult to sit in a chair, and the clinical setting seemed to cause him a lot of concern (Jane later found out he had a fear of hospitals). The young man's behaviour began to escalate to him swearing and shouting at Jane. He then picked up a chair and threatened to throw it at her. Jane used her Low Arousal training, which meant that she spoke very calmly and used non-verbal communication (holding her hands up and stepping back from the client). The client slammed the chair down on the ground, sat down and began to cry. Intuitively, she asked him whether she should leave the room to allow him time to calm down, or whether he wanted to leave the room for a moment. When the client indicated that he wanted her to stay, he began the process of calming down. The entire situation of escalation to de-escalation lasted no more than five minutes. She then carried on her task of getting health information from him without incident. Jane went on to develop a good working relationship with this person.

The above example moves us beyond guiding principles to a practical example of using Low Arousal approaches when someone is highly distressed and we do not know the causes. Jane very much focused on how she could calm down the individual in the moment. Low Arousal Approaches in this context meant Jane focusing on her non-verbal cues and keeping dialogue with this person to a minimum. By focusing on regulating her own behaviour, Jane created a calm, non-threatening response.

AN EXERCISE IN LOW AROUSAL

How we respond to situations can lead to either increasing or reducing arousal, as the following example shows:

> A hospital doctor was confronted with a drunk individual who required sutures. He was being observed by a student nurse in a small cubicle area with a curtain. The individual was clearly confused and distressed, and became verbally aggressive, swearing and shouting at individuals.

Imagine you are that student nurse: how can you help in this situation? Consider the following different response options:

1. Tell the person politely and firmly not to use abusive language in this setting
2. Call security to have the man physically held while his sutures are put in place, allowing him to be processed through the emergency department as rapidly as possible
3. Say nothing to the individual, and ignore his abusive language. Process him through the emergency department as rapidly as possible in order to reduce the distress to other people

---

Nonetheless, creating calm environments in healthcare settings can be challenging. Nurses are expected to work on hospital wards, outpatient clinics and in people's homes. In recent years in the NHS, waiting lists in general have tended to be longer, which often means that areas such as waiting rooms can become rapidly overcrowded (Appleby, 2022). Overcrowding has often been associated with increased hostility (Calhoun, 1962). It is important to think about the environment in busy hospitals and avoid 'hot spots' where distressed people are clustered together. Even relatively simple information such as telling people realistic timescales for how long they are expected to wait to see a healthcare professional can make a huge difference to people's behavioural responses (Nicholls, 2014). There is considerable research which even demonstrates that people can become 'calmer' by responding to the colours and hues in an environment (Elliot, 2015). Responding to people in environments such as these can be a challenging process, but it is important to remember that we can make a big difference by taking a reflective approach (McDonnell, 2019).

Often, the best Low Arousal response is to try and avoid inadvertently triggering and escalating the individual. Option 3 is the closest to a Low Arousal Approach, but it requires an individual to be tolerant and confident to manage the situation. A student nurse in this example should not consider themselves to be a completely passive observer of events. They are part of this social situation, and by exuding calmness and co-regulation can influence those around them. Whether option 1, 2 or 3 is chosen, it is important that people are allowed time to reflect and debrief.

Low Arousal Approaches can be highly effective in reducing conflict situations, but they also require us to view situations like these not in terms of a 'victim' and a 'perpetrator', but by seeing an individual who is stressed and traumatised, and acknowledging our own role in escalating crisis situations.

Conclusion

In the UK, guidelines have emerged in response to several exposés regarding the inhumane treatment of autistic people and individuals with a learning disability. Recent undercover documentaries, such as BBC *Panorama*'s 'Undercover Hospital Abuse Scandal' (2019), have exposed examples of degrading, inappropriate and inhumane use of restrictive practices. The author has been involved as an expert in a number of these televised documentaries about abuse in the care sector, including the notable Winterbourne View scandal (2011). The slippery slope to abuse often tells us that toxic cultures such as these emerge slowly over time (McDonnell et al., 2014). The Low Arousal Approaches described in this chapter are a practical set of tools that focus on respectful management of day-to-day behaviours, placing a positive focus on supporting individuals who may be distressed and traumatised.

All nurses are expected to manage distress in a range of environments, which will undoubtedly be a challenge for the nurses of today and in the future. Student nurses are the practitioners of tomorrow. Thinking about how we manage situations using conflict resolution methods such as Low Arousal Approaches will need to become a guiding principle in nursing practice. In this chapter, we have outlined the Low Arousal Approach to managing distressed behaviours and situations that often occur in healthcare environments. Student nurses are likely to encounter people who are distressed and witness some degree of 'challenging' behaviour throughout their training. The aim of this chapter is to allow the reader to reflect on how they respond to distressed behaviours. It is important to end on an optimistic note: whilst we could focus on factors that we cannot change quickly in the NHS, such as staffing, training, recruitment and government funding, we can control day-to-day issues by becoming experts at conflict resolution. The Low Arousal Approach will always encourage people to think about 'the here and now'. Becoming proficient in managing day-to-day conflict situations is a skill that we can all learn in order to become more confident practitioners. It is useful to remind people when they read about the Low Arousal Approach that it is essentially about changing our own behavioural responses to distressing situations. In essence, it is about 'us', not 'them'.

References

Anderson, C.A. & Bushman, B.J. (2002). Human aggression. *Annual Review of Psychology*, 53, 27–51.

Appleby, J. (2022). Chart of the week: How has the waiting list changed over the years? *Nuffield Trust* [Online]. Available from: https://www.nuffieldtrust.org.uk/resource/chart-of-the-week-how-has-the-waiting-list-changed-over-the-years.

Arik, C., Anat, R. & Arie, E. (2012). Encountering anger in the Emergency Department: Identification, evaluations and responses of staff members to anger displays. *Emergency Medicine International*, 2012(11): 603215. doi: 10.1155/2012/603215.

Beattie, J., Innes, K., Griffiths, D., & Morphet, J. (2020). Workplace violence: Examination of the tensions between duty of care, worker safety, and zero tolerance. *Health Care Management Review*, 45(3): E13–E22. doi: 10.1097/HMR.0000000000000286.

Calhoun, J.B. (1962). Population density and social pathology. *Scientific American*, 206, 139–148.

Cheung, K., Ching, S.S.Y, Cheng, S.H.N., & Ho, S.S.M. (2019). Prevalence and impact of clinical violence towards nursing students in Hong Kong: A cross-sectional study. *BMJ Open*, 9(5): e027385. doi: 10.1136/bmjopen-2018-027385.

Delahooke, M. (2019). *Beyond Behaviours: Using Brain Science and Compassion to Understand and Solve Children's Behavioral Challenges.* London: John Murray Press.

Desautels, L.L. (2020). *Connections Over Compliance: Rewiring Our Perceptions of Discipline.* Oregon: Wyatt-MacKenzie Publishing.

Elliot, A.J. (2015). Color and psychological functioning: A review of theoretical and empirical work. *Frontiers in Psychology*, 6: 1–8. doi: 10.3389/fpsyg.2015.00368.

Elvén, B.H. (2010). *No Fighting, No Biting, No Screaming: How to Make Behaving Positively Possible for People with Autism and Other Developmental Disabilities.* London: Jessica Kingsley Publishers

ICN, ICRC, IHF & WHO (2022). Violence Against Healthcare: Current Practices to Prevent, Reduce or Mitigate Violence Against Healthcare [Online]. Available from https://www.icn.ch/system/files/2022-07/Violence%20against%20healthcare%20survey%20report.pdf.

Lipsky, D. (2011). *From Anxiety to Meltdown: How Individuals on the Autism Spectrum Deal with Anxiety, Experience Meltdowns, Manifest Tantrums, and How You Can Intervene Effectively.* London: Jessica Kingsley Publishers.

Lundström, M., Aström, S. & Graneheim, U.H. (2007). Caregivers' experiences of exposure to violence in services for people with learning disabilities. *Journal of Psychiatric and Mental Health Nursing*, 14(4), 338–345. doi: 10.1111/j.1365-2850.2007.01081.x

McDonnell, A. (2019). *The Reflective Journey: A Practitioner's Guide to the Low Arousal Approach.* Peterborough: Studio 3 Publishing.

McDonnell, A. (2022) *Freedom from Restraint and Seclusion: The Studio 3 Approach.* Peterborough: Studio 3 Publishing.

McDonnell, A., Breen, E., Deveau, R., Goulding, E. & Smyth, J. (2014). How nurses and carers can avoid the slippery slope to abuse. *Learning Disability Practice*, 17(5): 36–39. doi: 10.7748/ldp.17.5.36.e1516.

McDonnell, A., McCreadie, M. & Dickinson, P. (2019). Behavioural issues and supports. In R. Jordan, J.M. Roberts & K. Hume (eds) *The SAGE Handbook of Autism and Education.* California: SAGE Publishing.

McDonnell, A., McEvoy, J. & Dearden, R.L. (1994). Coping with violent situations in the caring environment. In T. Wykes (ed.), *Violence and Health Care Professionals* (pp.189–206). Boston: Springer.

Nicholls, R. (2014). Managing patient-to-patient interaction: The waiting room experience. *University of Worcester* [Online]. Unpublished manuscript. Available from: https://eprints.worc.ac.uk/3818/3/Healthcare%2520and%2520patient%2520to%2520patient%2520interaction%2520R%2520Nicholls.pdf.

NMC. (2018). Future nurse: Standards of proficiency for registered nurses. Available at: future-nurse-proficiencies.pdf (nmc.org.uk)

Page, A., Elvén, B.H., Seabra, S., Warren, A., McDonnell, A., Mortiboys, I.L. & Vanes, N. (2019). Clinical holding: Ethical guidance for children's nurses working in the UK. *Nursing Children and Young People*, 31(4). doi: 10.7748/ncyp.2019.e1021.

Panorama. (2019). 'Undercover Hospital Abuse Scandal', BBC One.

Panorama. (2011). 'Undercover Care: The Abuse Exposed', BBC One.

Porges, S. W. (2011). *The Polyvagal Theory: Neurophysiological Foundations of Emotions, Attachment, Communication, and Self-regulation* (Norton Series on Interpersonal Neurobiology). New York: W.W. Norton & Company.

Swami, V. Hochstöger, S., Kargl, E. & Stieger, S. (2022). Hangry in the field: An experience sampling study on the impact of hunger on anger, irritability, and affect. *PLOS ONE.* doi: 10.1371/journal.pone.0269629.

Swift, J. (2003). *Gulliver's Travels.* London: Penguin Books. (Original work published 1726.)

Vuolo, J.C. (2017). Student nurses' experiences of incivility and the impact on learning and emotional wellbeing. *Journal of Nursing Education and Practice*, 8(4): 102–111. doi: 10.5430/jnep.v8n4p102.

Woodcock, L. & Page A. (2010). *Manging Family Meltdown: The Low Arousal Approach and Autism.* London: Jessica Kingsley Publishers.

Conditions that all nurses and allied health professionals need to be aware of in people with learning disabilities

Ruth Hirst, Sheryl King and Victoria Moloney

Introduction

This chapter will explore three common health diagnoses which are recognised in LeDeR (Learning from Lives and Deaths of People with Learning Disabilities and Autism) reviews (NHS, n.d.; NHS England, 2017; King's College London, 2021, 2022) as contributing to the death in people with learning disabilities and autism. Reviews into the deaths of this population are extensive with the first report from Mencap's Death by Indifference (2007) followed by Confidential Inquiry into Premature Deaths of People with Learning Disabilities (CIPOLD) (2013) and culminating with the most recent report from LeDeR in 2022 which shows a drop in avoidable deaths from 50% in 2021 to 42% in avoidable deaths in 2022 (King's College London, 2023). The three common health diagnoses are: constipation, gastro-oesophageal reflux disorder (GORD) and sepsis.

The Foreword from Paula McGowan OBE at the beginning of this book highlights the ongoing need for anyone working with people with a learning disability and/or autism to be competent, knowledgeable and compassionate in their holistic support of the person. We know that people with a learning disability experience poorer health outcomes than the general population with several inquiries identifying that they are more likely to die from treatable causes (NHS England, 2018).

The following themes are not exhaustive; however, they should always be considered and implemented across all inpatients, outpatients and community health settings. Be aware that not everyone will have a formal diagnosis of learning disability and/or those with a mild learning disability are unlikely to have a hospital passport or support services in situ.

- If in a GP, social care or hospital setting be aware that this person may have an alert on their records which details a learning disability along with any

DOI: 10.4324/9781003341765-16

safeguarding concerns (NHS England, 2023). Please note that each alert is individual to the system used by the organisation.

■ Is there a risk of diagnostic overshadowing? The RCN (2021) describes this occurring 'when a health professional makes the assumption that the behaviour of a person with learning disabilities is part of their disability without exploring other factors such as biological determinants'.

■ Ensuring reasonable adjustments (Equality Act 2010) are considered and applied.

■ Mental Capacity Act 2005 – people with learning disabilities should be deemed as having capacity unless assessed otherwise.

■ Importance of initial assessment.

■ Finding out when was the last annual health check – current medication, allergies.

■ Do they have a hospital passport and has it been read?

■ Importance of joined-up working/collaboration – what team is the individual under, are the acute liaison nurses involved?

■ Factoring in transition (child to adult) if a young person.

■ Understanding how the individual communicates so they can be part of any health decisions made with/about them.

Behaviour

Much has been written about people with learning disabilities and autism and 'challenging behaviour'. Unfortunately, this term is often misused as a form of diagnosis despite it *not* being identified as one under the International Classification of Diseases (ICD11). The term 'challenging behaviour' is itself a barrier to people with a learning disability accessing healthcare services as once this appears in their notes it can mean that healthcare professionals do not treat them as they would the general population, leading to missed opportunities to meet their needs appropriately by diagnostic overshadowing. Think of changes in behaviour as distressed and/or communicative – they are telling you something is wrong but may not be able to verbally explain this to you in what we would consider 'appropriate ways'. Peebles and Price (2011) stated that self-injurious behaviours may be used as a coping strategy if the pain area is difficult to identify. Therefore, when working with individuals with a learning disability, if you are told that there has been a behaviour change instead of blaming their diagnosis please listen and conduct further tests to rule out any physical causes.

Health conditions

There are many common health conditions experienced by individuals with a learning disability. However, their presentation may differ from the general population, including:

■ Respiratory

■ Epilepsy

- Cardiac
- Cancers
- Oral health

For the purposes of this chapter the focus will be on:

- Constipation/bowel health
- GORD (gastro-oesophageal reflux disease)
- Sepsis

This is because in the 2022 LeDeR report (KCL, 2023) these three health conditions were in the top ten conditions leading to causes of death. NHS England and NHS Improvement (NHSE and NHSI, 2020) released their report, *Quality Improvement Domain 2020/21 – Supporting People with Learning Disabilities*, which stated that constipation and GORD alongside obesity, asthma, dysphagia, epilepsy, dementia and mental health problems are the more common health co-morbidities for people with learning disabilities.

Constipation

Brief overview:

- 2013: In the *Confidential Inquiry into Premature Deaths of People with Learning Disabilities*, constipation was one of the most frequently reported health conditions deemed treatable amongst people with a learning disability (Heslop et al., 2013).

- 2013: McCarron et al. (2013) identified that individuals with a learning disability are a population more at risk of developing health issues than the general population with constipation being a common gastrointestinal condition experienced.

- 2016: Public Health England (PHE) (2016) state individuals with a learning disability have a higher prevalence of constipation than the general population.

- 2018: Individuals with a learning disability are at increased risk of constipation due to specific medications they are likely to be prescribed that cause the side effect of constipation. Further to this, individuals with a learning disability are at a higher risk of living a sedentary lifestyle including poor diet, limited exercise and mobility (Robertson et al., 2018).

- 2019: In the *Learning from Lives and Deaths (LeDeR)* 2019 report it was identified that constipation was a top five common health condition in the deaths of individuals with a learning disability.

- 2021: In the *Learning from Lives and Deaths (LeDeR)* 2021 report constipation was not included in the top 14 common health condition despite the risk of complications and possible death if left undetected.

- 2023: NHS England (2023) in conjunction with those with lived experience launched a campaign to develop constipation resources for those working in primary care services, to support individuals with a learning disability around the detection, prevention and treatment of constipation.

■ 2023: In the *Learning from Lives and Deaths (LeDeR)* 2022 report, constipation was included as one of the top 12 common health conditions and was identified as a priority area to be explored for future policy planning.

Constipation and people with learning disabilities

Constipation is a common health condition that can affect people across the lifespan (NICE, 2024a). Symptoms include difficulty or infrequency in passing stools, hard stools and feeling of unfinished emptying of the bowel (Bharucha, Pemberton and Locke, 2013). It is experienced and treated as a short-term condition as it is considered preventable; however, it can be a much longer-term condition (Public Health England, 2016). Robertson et al. (2018) suggest that it should be an active diagnosis due to the serious implications on health and quality of life.

Constipation is a condition more likely to be experienced by individuals with a learning disability than in the general population (Robertson et al., 2018). The condition can be identified and managed in the community, but often leads to hospital admission (Glover & Evison, 2013). The condition poses a significant risk to health including death in people with a learning disability as symptoms may be missed if support in communicating these are not in place (Pouard, 2023).

Causes and risk factors of constipation in individuals with a learning disability
Co-morbidities and associated syndromes with learning disability

■ Co-morbidities such as epilepsy, anxiety, depression, obesity and diabetes (PHE, 2016).

■ Individuals with severe to profound learning disability and physical disability including cerebral palsy, reduced mobility, postural issues and dysphagia (Laugharne et al., 2024; Robertson et al., 2018).

■ Individuals with Down syndrome experiencing associated conditions hypothyroidism and/or Hirschsprung's disease (NICE, 2024b).

Medication

■ Likely to be prescribed anti-psychotics, anti-depressants, anticonvulsants and opium which cause side effects of constipation (Robertson et al., 2018; McMahon et al., 2020; Laugharne et al., 2024).

■ Increased use of laxatives and risk of laxative polypharmacy for management and prevention of constipation (Robertson et al., 2018; AlMutairi et al., 2020).

Sedentary lifestyle

■ Contributory factors associated with individuals with a learning disability experiencing constipation include poor diet and limited fluid intake/dehydration, limited exercise and limited mobility (Horan et al., 2020).

- Likely to have lower intake of fruit and vegetables leading to low-fibre diet (Public Health England, 2016).

Social and lifestyle

- Limited education and lack of understanding of the need to defecate and how to go to the toilet (Bladder and Bowel UK, 2017).

- Communication barriers when experiencing symptoms, reliance on carers and reluctance to report need to use the toilet (Maslen et al., 2022; Pouard, 2023).

- Lack of facilities and privacy (Pouard, 2023).

- Increased anxiety (Public Health England, 2016).

Complications of these – what can you do?

- Can lead to death if not addressed (King's College London, 2019; Inquest, 2018).

- Chronic constipation, faecal incontinence and faecal impaction (PHE, 2016).

- Can lead to diagnostic overshadowing and vital symptoms being missed (Maslen et al, 2022; Marsh and McMeel, 2023).

- Reduced quality of life (Public Health England, 2016).

TABLE 14.1 Presentation

Typical presentation for constipation	Things to be aware of if the person has a learning disability
Abdominal pain, cramps and/or bloating, diarrhoea	Distended abdomen, changes in bowel pattern and type, vomiting, difficulty passing stools, faecal overflow due to constipation and partial obstruction, twisting of the bowel, spending longer periods of time in the toilet. Rectal bleeding which may result in anal fissures, haemorrhoids or rectal prolapse (Horan et al., 2020; Public Health England, 2016)
Loss of appetite or nausea	Potential weight loss, eating less, check if reduced fibre in diet, headaches, drinking less, signs of dehydration – dry mouth, oral mucosa, sunken eyes, dry and/or cool skin (Public Health England, 2016; Horan et al., 2020)
Affects sleep and daily living activities	Disturbed sleep due to bloating and pain, caffeine intake and timing (Horan et al., 2020)
Affects mental health – anxiety, embarrassment, social isolation, distress	Changes in mood, heightened anxiety, agitation, withdrawn, depression (Public Health England, 2016)
Behavioural symptoms	Aggression, self-harm, self-injury such as rectal digging, sensory processing and interoception of elimination, pain, itch (Public Health England, 2016; Marsh and McMeel, 2023)

- Signs and symptoms could lead to potentially more serious conditions including cancer, ulcerative colitis, irritable bowel syndrome (NICE, 2024b).

See 'Treatment, resources and actions' on what you can do for prevention and effective management of constipation in individuals with a learning disability.

Gastro-oesophageal reflux disease (GORD)

Brief overview

Gastro-oesophageal reflux disorder (GORD) is often described using the Montreal definition which states it develops when the reflux of stomach contents causes troublesome symptoms and/or complications (Schneider, 2007; Ronkainen & Agréus, 2013; Nirwan et al., 2020; Howard et al., 2023).

GORD is one of the most common physical complaints for people with learning disabilities (Simpson, Mizen and Cooper, 2020). It can be a debilitating and lifelong condition requiring long-term use of medication, lifestyle changes and possible surgery to manage (Howard et al., 2023; Nirwan et al., 2020).

GORD more commonly impacts on both children and adults with neurological conditions such as learning disabilities and cerebral palsy, whereas in the general population it is seen more in adults (Howard et al., 2023).

Diseases of the digestive system (including GORD) are within the ten top causes of death for people with learning disabilities as reported by LeDeR (2021) with it relating to 6% of deaths in 2021; a rise of 0.5% from 2020 but a drop from 7.2% (2018) and 6.7% (2019).

GORD can also impact on oral health and respiratory diseases due to aspiration as well as links to dysphagia of which more deaths have been reported to LeDeR (KCL, 2023) as a cause. GORD is also associated as a risk factor for endocrine, nutritional and metabolic diseases which is also in the ten most common causes of death for people with learning disabilities (Nomura et al., 2014).

GORD has a higher prevalence in individuals with a learning disability/neuro-disabilities because it is overlooked as a diagnosis when clinicians are faced with behaviours; and are instead linked to the individual's neurological diagnosis as opposed to a physical cause leading to diagnostic overshadowing (Simpson, Mizen and Cooper, 2020).

Sanna et al. (2013) reviewed the link between GORD and increased likelihood of anxiety, depression and distressed states. People with learning disabilities are more likely to present as distressed without being able to verbalise what is wrong and therefore using a tool such as DisDAT (Distress and Discomfort Assessment Tool) to understand the causes and the individual's communication of distress may be beneficial to rule out diagnostic overshadowing (Regnard et al., 2007).

GORD in people with learning disabilities is linked to further complications due to later diagnosis (Peebles and Price, 2011).

Complications of these, what can you do?

- Consider the impact on health-related quality of life for the person.

TABLE 14.2 Presentation

GORD	Things to be aware of if the person has a learning disability
Heart burn – chest pain but not cardiac related, especially after eating	The person may cry after eating, may present as hitting themselves on their chest, rubbing their neck, hand mouthing (Peebles and Price, 2011).
Acid reflux – where stomach acid comes back up into your mouth and causes an unpleasant, sour taste	Spitting, drooling, retching
Rumination – regurgitating food and rechewing partially	Chewing motion, spitting food out, excessive swallowing
Silent reflux: Hoarseness to voice, coughing, choking episodes (especially at night), dry throat, feeling like there's something stuck in their throat	May see more throat clearing, coughing and nighttime choking incidences.
Oesophagitis (a sore, inflamed oesophagus)	A hoarse cry, crying on swallowing, holding food or drink in their mouth for longer as it hurts to swallow
Bad breath, tooth decay/erosion and gum disease	It is so important that dental appointments are carried out as, due to silent reflux and for those with limited communication, this is often the first time it will be picked up (Howard et al, 2023).
Bloating and belching	Excessive belching, not wanting to eat or drink therefore pushing items away or not touching them – we should always investigate if there is a change in their eating and drinking habits
Feeling or being sick	Behaviours – spitting, hitting themselves/others, regurgitation, crying
Pain when swallowing or difficulty on swallowing	Crying, holding throat, rubbing ears or hitting side of head
Sore throat, hoarseness or persistent cough/hiccup which may be worse at night	Can also be linked to increase in behaviours, frustration, crying out, hitting self and behaviours noted in above sections. A persistent cough has been linked to micro-aspirations which can take place day or night, which may not respond to PPIs (Niimi, 2017).

- Oesophageal erosion especially if silent reflux is present – long-term acid can lead to more serious complications such as Barrett's Oesophagus which is a change in the oesophageal cells due to heartburn and acid reflux and can potentially lead to cancer developing (Parasa and Sharma, 2013).

- H.Pylori factors to consider – NICE (2019) guidance on GORD states doing testing to rule this out when assessing and diagnosing GORD and complications; this is due to H.Pylori increasing the risk of GORD as well as cancer (Harper et al., 2020). However, Parasa and Sharma (2013) state there is a decreasing prevalence of H.Pylori.

- Obesity can be a contributing factor to the development of GORD due to increased intra-abdominal pressure and risk of developing hiatus hernias (Ronkainen, 2013).

- Oral health may be impacted by GORD and can be a contributing factor to poor dental hygiene (Lechien et al., 2020; Hartnett and McNamara, 2021; Howard et al., 2023).

- In older people there may be multiple comorbidities resulting in a range of medications and potential contraindications (AlMutairi et al., 2018).

- Aspiration – silent reflux or regurgitation of foods which may then pass into the airways carry complications such pneumonia and infection (Niimi, 2017).

Treatment: adjustments to the person, need for reviews:

- See past the behaviour and commence physical health checks early.

- The use of Proton Pump Inhibitors (PPIs) has been researched and shown to reduce behaviours that may be deemed as challenging due to treating the underlying cause (Peebles and Price, 2011) and using the lowest effective dose to manage symptoms once symptoms are under control (Pratt et al., 2016).

- Ask when the last annual health check occurred and if it has not been completed to get this booked.

- Work with the person, family and other HCPs involved in the care of the individual as they will have a good understanding of how they usually present and any changes i.e. a time scale of changes happening.

- Use of PPIs such as Omeprazole to manage and reduce symptoms.

- Long-term diet/lifestyle changes – ensuring the individual is involved in this and understands the reasons why therefore using easy read information/social stories to explain what is happening.

- NICE (2019) guidance on GORD and dyspepsia states that patients with a GORD diagnosis should have annual health reviews; this would coincide with the annual health checks for people with learning disabilities carried out by GPs from the age of 14 years old.

Sepsis

Brief overview

- 2013: Incidence and mortality rates of sepsis increasing dramatically with similar incidence to heart attack and mortality rate similar to lung cancer, with each hospital admission costing approximately £20,000 (PHSO 2013).

- 2016–2017 LeDeR Annual report recorded 11% deaths as sepsis related whilst also reporting sepsis to be third most common cause of death for people with a learning disability in 2016 (LeDeR, 2017).

- 2017: World Health Organization (WHO) made sepsis a global priority (WHO, 2017).

- 2020: Most of the recommendations from the LeDeR Annual Report (2020) where sepsis was identified as a cause of death focused upon the need for training for families and paid carers on infection prevention and recognition of early warning signs plus training for healthcare professionals on the provision of reasonable adjustment for people with learning disabilities.

About sepsis and people with learning disabilities

Sepsis is a serious life-threatening condition characterised by the body's immune system having an extreme response to a bacterial infection or other viral, parasitic or fungal infection, affecting millions of people worldwide every year (WHO, 2023). The NHS Long Term Plan (2019) identifies that in England sepsis is responsible for the loss of 37,000 lives a year and that every NHS Trust must act to identify and treat this condition.

The most common triggers for sepsis are lower respiratory tract or urine infections and people with a learning disability are five times more likely to be admitted to hospital with such infections compared to people without a learning disability (Hunt and Harding, 2019). Linked with these are other factors including swallowing difficulties putting individuals at greater risk of aspiration and becoming frail at a younger age (Foster, 2021).

About 80% of hospital-treated sepsis cases originate from community acquired infection (Cecconi et al., 2018). This has implications for people with learning disability who live in the community in places of multiple occupancy whether in a family home, residential setting or supported living accommodation. A very recent and first nationwide study conducted by Zhong et al. (2023) into links between health inequalities and community acquired non-Covid sepsis found that certain clinical factors increased this risk which included having a learning disability. Sepsis can also develop as a consequence of Covid-19 (UK Sepsis Trust n.d.). This is particularly pertinent to people with learning disabilities who in England were reported to have the highest death rate from Covid-19 because of poor support (Taggart et al., 2022).

Early deterioration in physical health is key to optimum recovery and survival of sepsis but for people with a learning disability this is impacted by diagnostic overshadowing, an inability to recognise, understand and communicate symptoms on the part of the individual, a lack of training/education for carers, capacity and accessibility issues with being examined. Therefore, people with a learning disability have higher rates of co-morbid health conditions and compared to the general population are three to four times as likely to die from an avoidable medical cause of death (NICE, 2021). Hence, the early identification of ill health in this population of people is vital along with ensuring that assumptions are not made and that all abnormal observations (vital signs or otherwise) are responded to.

Sepsis is a time critical condition. Curiosity is key to early signs of infection which can be grouped into: chest infections where the person has a cough, shortness of breath, urine infections where there is pain or frequency on passing urine or loin pain. Gastrointestinal infections may present as abdominal pain, diarrhoea

TABLE 14.3 Presentation: sepsis 6 in adults – the danger signs where emergency action is needed

Sepsis 6	Things to be aware of if person has a learning disability
Slurred speech/confusion/ decline in functional skills	Recognition of new onset confusion. Evidence of a change in mental and functional state from 'normal' baseline. This person may already have slurred speech or even no audible speech therefore behavioural observations and careful history taking is important. Awareness of usual communication methods needed
Extreme shivering or muscle pain	Person may not be able to communicate pain verbally but may express it through facial expressions, bodily movements and behaviours of concern There may be visible shivering or shaking of body
Passing no urine (in a day) or reduced urine output/ raised heart rate	A person may be incontinent and reliant upon the use of incontinence products so ensure observation of absorbency levels. Awareness of someone who is catheterised and careful recording of urinary output and fluid intake.
Severe breathlessness/ raised respiratory rate/ hypotension	Respiratory distress even if sitting still Consider the baseline of respiratory rate for the individual as this is likely to vary due to various factors including severity of learning disability and the health conditions
It feels like you're going to die	The person may not recognise or articulate such a feeling but may present with confusion, anxiety, fear, dysregulated behaviour Having a very fast heartbeat
Skin mottled or discoloured/ pallor/cyanosed skin, lips or tongue/any rash	Compromised skin integrity or signs of infection. There may be a history of self-injurious behaviour with lesions not healed. * In people with Down syndrome this may be missed as skin does not mottle

or vomiting and wound infections can present as broken skin that is red, tender with or without discharge. A fever may also be present where there is infection. It is in these early stages that advice should be sought from an individual's GP or an NHS 111 where it should be made clear that there is a concern that sepsis is may be evident.

Treatment, resources and actions for working with any individuals with a learning disability for constipation, sepsis and GORD or other health conditions

- ■ Knowledge and understanding – educating those that support the person, staff/ carer training.

- ■ Liaising with the individual, family and carers – they know the individual and can advise on changes and timelines of events. They also know how to best communicate with the person.

- ■ Healthcare professionals having the awareness and understanding of how people with learning disabilities may present to enable high-quality care.

TABLE 14.4 Additional considerations on treatment, resources and actions for each health condition

Constipation	Sepsis	GORD
• Use simple, well-known terminology • Use Bristol Stool Chart/diary to monitor stools • Bowel monitoring and knowing what is normal for the person • Consistency in care and support for the person • Education on toileting including how to use the toilet, have effective bowel movements, balanced diet and promote good posture • Use of diet monitoring charts including tracking fluid and fibre intake • Medication monitoring and regular reviews under STOMP (NHS England, 2016) • Observe physical and mental health changes	Use SBAR when communicating with emergency services/GP concerns that sepsis might be suspected. For example: Situation Check me for Sepsis Song: https://www.youtube.com/watch?v=FZq5sYulOB8 to raise awareness & improve vigilance to the signs of sepsis amongst people with a learning disability (Purple All Stars, 2019) Sepsis information for paid carers/professionals of people with a learning disability: https://www.youtube.com/watch?v=KPY6tLgmChE (Sherwood Forest Hospitals, 2019) Podcast on recognising deterioration and sepsis in people with a learning disability. https://www.e-lfh.org.uk/wp-content/uploads/2021/06/sepsis-podcast-audio-oct-2020.mp3 (NHS England, eLearning for healthcare, 2020)	• Regular dental health checks are important as this can be when GORD may first be identified • Monitoring any changes to or new behaviours around eating and drinking • Use of Omeprazole or other PPIs to manage/reduce symptoms as this can also improve behaviours associated with the diagnosis but which may be labelled as 'challenging'

■ Reasonable adjustments to be made such as use of easy-read and accessible information.

■ Hospital passport, annual health checks, health action plans – having access to these across healthcare teams, e.g. GPs, hospitals.

■ Use of the DisDAT: Distress and Discomfort Assessment Tool to identify reasons for changes to presentation.

■ Functional analysis screening tool (FAST) to again identify changes to behaviour.

■ Initial assessment: important to consider physical health and not focus on behaviours which may be challenging but find out what might be causing them.

Conclusion and key points

The information in this chapter is based upon recent and historical evidence that highlights the significant health inequalities experienced by individuals with a learning disability. The three health conditions discussed each present differently in this population therefore conventional approaches may need adaptation to meet individual need. Creativity is required by every health professional who has contact with individuals with a learning disability as part of their legal responsibility to practise within the Equality Act 2010 and The Mental Capacity Act 2005.

- Collaboration is key to improve healthcare for individuals with learning disabilities. Do not work in a silo.

- Reflect on your attitude to a person's diagnosis, see the person not the diagnosis.

- Remember: health passports are your passport to understanding the whole person.

References

AlMutairi, H., O'Dwyer, M., Burke, E., McCarron, M., McCallion, P. and Henman, M.C. (2020). Laxative use among older adults with intellectual disability: A cross-sectional observational study. *International Journal of Clinical Pharmacy*, 42, pp. 89–99. doi: https://doi.org/10.1007/s11096-019-00942-z

AlMutairi, H., O'Dwyer, M., McCarron, M., McCallion, P. and Henman, M.C. (2018). The use of proton pump inhibitors among older adults with intellectual disability: A cross sectional observational study. *Saudi Pharmaceutical Journal*, 26(7), pp. 1012–1021. doi: https://doi.org/10.1016/j.jsps.2018.05.009

Bharucha, A. E., Pemberton, J. H., & Locke III, G. R. (2013). American Gastroenterological Association technical review on constipation. *Gastroenterology*, 144(1), pp. 218–238. https://doi.org/10.1053/j.gastro.2012.10.028

Bladder and Bowel UK (2017). Constipation in people with learning difficulties. [online] Available at: https://www.bbuk.org.uk/wp-content/uploads/2021/02/Understanding-constipation-in-people-with-learning-difficulties.pdf [Accessed 02/05/2024]

Brown, M., Surfraz, M., Wroldsen, R., Popa, D. and Grung, R.-M. (2017). Improving healthcare access for people with intellectual disabilities in four European countries. *Learning Disability Practice*, 20(6), pp. 36–42. doi: https://doi.org/10.7748/ldp.2017.e1873

Cecconi, M., Evans, L., Levy, M. and Rhodes, A. (2018). Sepsis and septic shock. *The Lancet*, 392(10141), pp. 75–87. https://doi-org.bcu.idm.oclc.org/10.1016/S0140-6736(18)30696-2

Charlot, L., Abend, S., Ravin, P., Mastis, K., Hunt, A. and Deutsch, C. (2010). Non-psychiatric health problems among psychiatric inpatients with intellectual disabilities. *Journal of Intellectual Disability Research*, 55(2), pp. 199–209. doi: https://doi.org/10.1111/j.1365-2788.2010.01294.x [Accessed 05.09.2023]

Doherty, P., Barksby, J. and McCorkindale, M. (2021). Signs and symptoms of sepsis: Raising awareness in the learning disability community. *Learning Disability Practice*, 24(2), pp. 27–32. doi: https://doi.org/10.7748/ldp.2021.e2099.

Easy Health. (n.d.). *Gastro-Oesophageal Reflux Disorder (GORD)*. [online] Available at: https://www.easyhealth.org.uk/pages/16-gastro-oesophageal-reflux-disorder-gord [Accessed 16 October 2023]

Foster, M. (2021). Raising awareness of the signs and symptoms of sepsis in people with a learning disability. Available at: https://www.governmentevents.co.uk/wp-content/uploads/2021/09/Sepsis-Conference-7.9.21-Learning-Disability-Sepsis.pdf. [Accessed 30.11.2023]

Glover, G. and Evison, F. (2013). Hospital admissions that should not happen: Admissions for ambulatory care sensitive conditions for people with learning disabilities in England:

Improving health & lives. *Learning Disabilities Observatory*. Available at: https://www.ihal. org.uk/gsf.php5?f= 16714 [Accessed 21/12/2023]

Grant, N., Hewitt, O., Ash, K. and Knott, F. (2021). The experiences of sepsis in people with a learning disability – a qualitative investigation. *British Journal of Learning Disabilities*, 50(4), pp. 514–524. https://doi.org/10.1111/bld.12416

Harper, L., Boulter, P., Ambridge, A., Griffin, P. and Ooms, A. (2020). Helicobacter pylori: Nurses' perceptions of diagnosis and treatment in adults. *Learning Disability Practice*, 23(2), pp. 38–45. doi: https://doi.org/10.7748/ldp.2020.e2015

Hartnett, L. and McNamara, M. (2021). Oral health and supporting people with intellectual disabilities to get access to dental treatment. *Learning Disability Practice*, 24(2), pp. 33–41. doi: https://doi.org/10.7748/ldp.2021.e2123.

Heslop, P., Blair, P.S., Fleming, P., Hoghton, M., Marriott, A. and Russ, L. (2013). The Confidential Inquiry into premature deaths of people with intellectual disabilities in the UK: a population-based study. *The Lancet*, 383(9920), pp. 889–895.

Horan, P., Cleary, M., Fleming, S., Mulhere, J., Doyle, C., Burke, E., Byrne, K. and Keenan, P. (2020). Preventing, assessing and managing constipation in people with intellectual disabilities. *Learning Disability Practice*, 23(5), pp. 17–23. doi: https://doi.org/10.7748/ldp.2020. e2067.

Howard, J.P., Howard, L.J., Geraghty, J., A. Johanna Leven and Ashley, M. (2023). Gastrointestinal conditions related to tooth wear, 234(6), pp. 451–454. doi: https://doi. org/10.1038/s41415-023-5677-0.

Hunt, A. and Harding, K. (2019). 'Check me for sepsis, that's all I ask'. *Emergency Nurse*, 27(5), p.11.https://web.p.ebscohost.com/ehost/pdfviewer/pdfviewer?vid=0&sid=4443322d-691e-44dd-9180-37c3c3bd7b3d%40redis

Inquest (2018). Inquest into the premature death of Richard Handley identifies gross failures in care. [online]. Available at: https://www.inquest.org.uk/richard-handley-conclusion [Accessed 02/05/2024]

King's College London (2021). *Learning from Lives and Deaths People with a Learning Disability and Autistic People (LeDeR)*. [online] www.kcl.ac.uk. Available at: https://www.kcl.ac.uk/ research/leder [Accessed 01.08.2023]

King's College London (2022). *2022 LeDeR Report into the Avoidable Deaths of People with Learning Disabilities*. [online] King's College London. Available at: *https://www.kcl.ac.uk/news/2022-leder-report-into-the-avoidable-deaths-of-people-with-learning-disabilities*. [Accessed 13/02/2024]

Laugharne, R., Sawhney, I., Perera, B., Wainwright, D., Bassett, P., Caffrey, B., O'Dwyer, M., Lamb, K., Wilcock, M., Roy, A. and Oak, K. (2024). Chronic constipation in people with intellectual disabilities in the community: cross-sectional study. *BJPsych Open*, 10(2), p. e55. doi: https://doi.org/10.1192/bjo.2024.12

Lechien, J.R., Chiesa-Estomba, C.M., Calvo Henriquez, C., Mouawad, F., Ristagno, C., Barillari, M.R., Schindler, A., Nacci, A., Bouland, C., Laino, L. and Saussez, S. (2020). Laryngopharyngeal reflux, gastroesophageal reflux and dental disorders: A systematic review. *PLOS ONE*, 15(8), p. e0237581. doi: https://doi.org/10.1371/journal.pone.0237581

Marsh, L. and McMeel, A. (2023). How to support the accurate diagnosis of constipation in people with learning disabilities. *Learning Disability Practice*, 26(6). doi: https://doi. org/10.7748/ldp.2023.e2231

Maslen, C., Hodge, R., Tie, K., Laugharne, R., Lamb, K. and Shankar, R. (2022). Constipation in autistic people and people with learning disabilities. *British Journal of General Practice*, 72(720), pp. 348–351. doi: https://doi.org/10.3399/bjgp22x720077

McCarron, M., Swinburne, J., Burke, E., McGlinchey, E., Carroll, R. & McCallion, P. (2013). Patterns of multimorbidity in an older population of persons with an intellectual disability: results from the intellectual disability supplement to the Irish longitudinal study on aging (IDS-TILDA). Research in Developmental Disabilities, 34(1), 521–527.

McMahon M., Hatton C. and Bowring D. L. (2020). Polypharmacy and psychotropic polyphar-macy in adults with intellectual disability: A cross-sectional total population study. *Journal of Intellectual Disability Research*, 64(11), pp. 834–851. doi: https://doi.org/10.1111/jir.12775

NHS (n.d.). LeDeR Home. [online] Available at: https://leder.nhs.uk/ [Accessed 01.08.2023]

NHS England (2016). Stopping over medication of people with a learning disability, autism or both (STOMP). [online] Available at: https://www.england.nhs.uk/learning-disabilities/improving-health/stomp/ [Accessed 02/05/2024]

NHS England (2017). The Learning Disability Mortality Review Programme Annual Report. Available at: https://leder.nhs.uk/images/annual_reports/leder_annual_report_2016_2017.pdf

NHS England (2018). NHS England: The learning disability improvement standards for NHS trusts. [online] Available at: https://www.england.nhs.uk/learning-disabilities/about/resources/the-learning-disability-improvement-standards-for-nhs-trusts/. [Accessed 09.02.2023]

NHS England (2019). The NHS Long Term Plan to reduce toll of 'hidden killer' sepsis. Availableat:https://www.england.nhs.uk/2019/03/nhs-long-term-plan-to-reduce-toll-of-hidden-killer-sepsis/ [Accessed 24/11/2023]

NHS England (2020). The Learning Disabilities Mortality Review Programme Annual Report. Available at: LeDeR-bristol-annual-report-2020.pdf (england.nhs.uk)

NHS England (2023). Safeguarding. [online] Available at: https://www.england.nhs.uk/long-read/safeguarding/#:~:text=Alerts%20are%20routinely%20applied%20to [Accessed 9/02/2024]

NHSE and NHSI (2020). QOF Quality Improvement domain 2020/21 – Supporting people with learning disabilities. Available at: https://www.england.nhs.uk/wp-content/uploads/2020/02/20-21-qof-qi-supporting-people-with-learning-disabilites.pdf [Accessed 9/02/2024]

NHS England (2021). Learning from lives and deaths – People with a learning disability and autistic people (LeDeR) policy 2021. (online) Available at: https://www.england.nhs.uk/wp-content/uploads/2021/03/B0428-LeDeR-policy-2021.pdf [Accessed 01.08.2023]

NHS England, eLearning for healthcare (2020). Recognising deterioration & sepsis in people with a learning disability. [podcast] Available at: https://www.e-lfh.org.uk/wp-content/uploads/2021/06/sepsis-podcast-audio-oct-2020.mp3 [Accessed 09/02/2024]

NICE (National Institute for Health and Care Excellence) (2017). Risk Stratification tool for adults, children and YP aged 12 yrs and over with suspected sepsis. https://www.nice.org.uk/guidance/ng51/resources/table-1-risk-stratification-tool-for-adults-children-and-young-people-aged-12-years-and-over-with-suspected-sepsis-2551487005

NICE (National Institute for Health and Care Excellence) (2019). 2019 surveillance of gastro-oesophageal reflux disease and dyspepsia in adults: investigation and management (NICE guideline CG184). Available at: https://www.nice.org.uk/guidance/cg184/resources/2019-surveillance-of-gastrooesophageal-reflux-disease-and-dyspepsia-in-adults-investi-gation-and-management-nice-guideline-cg184-pdf-8639830448629

NICE (National Institute for Health and Care Excellence) (2020a). CKS is only available in the UK. [online] NICE. Available at: https://cks.nice.org.uk/topics/sepsis/background-information/risk-factors/ [Accessed 13.11.2023]

NICE (National Institute for Health and Care Excellence) (2020b). How should I assess a per-son with suspected sepsis? https://cks.nice.org.uk/topics/sepsis/diagnosis/assessment/

NICE (National Institute for Health and Care Excellence) (2021). NICE impact people with a learning disability. Available at: https://acppld.csp.org.uk/system/files/documents/2021-11/NICE%20Learning%20disability%20impact%20report.pdf [Accessed 30.11.2023]

nidirect.gov.uk. (2017). Heartburn and gastro-oesophageal reflux disease (GORD). nidirect. [online] Available at: https://www.nidirect.gov.uk/conditions/heartburn-and-gastro-oesophageal-reflux-disease-gord#:~:text=Gastro%2Doesophageal%20reflux%20dis-ease%20(GORD)%20is%20a%20common%20condition [Accessed 16.10.2023]

NICE (National Institute for Health and Care Excellence) (2024a). Constipation [online] Available at: https://cks.nice.org.uk/topics/constipation/ [Accessed 02.05.2024]

NICE (National Institute for Health and Care Excellence) (2024b). Constipation: What are the secondary causes? [online] Available at: https://cks.nice.org.uk/topics/constipation/background-information/secondary-causes/[Accessed 01.05.2024]

Niimi, A. (2017). Cough associated with gastro-oesophageal reflux disease (GORD): Japanese experience. *Pulmonary Pharmacology & Therapeutics*, 47, pp. 59–65. doi: https://doi.org/10.1016/j.pupt.2017.05.006.

Nirwan, J.S., Hasan, S.S., Babar, Z.-U.-D., Conway, B.R. and Ghori, M.U. (2020). Global prevalence and risk factors of gastro-oesophageal reflux disease (GORD): Systematic review with meta-analysis. *Scientific Reports*, [online] 10(1). doi: https://doi.org/10.1038/s41598-020-62795-1

Nomura, M., Tashiro, N., Watanabe, T., Hirata, A., Abe, I., Okabe, T. and Takayanagi, R. (2014). Association of symptoms of gastroesophageal reflux with metabolic syndrome parameters in patients with endocrine disease. *ISRN Gastroenterology*, 2014, pp. 1–6. doi: https://doi.org/10.1155/2014/863206

Parliamentary and Health Service Ombudsman (2013). Time to Act, Severe sepsis: rapid diagnosis and treatment saves lives. Available at: https://www.ombudsman.org.uk/sites/default/files/Time_to_act_report.pdf [Accessed 24/11/2023]

Parasa, S. and Sharma, P. (2013). Complications of gastro-oesophageal reflux disease. *Best Practice & Research Clinical Gastroenterology*, 27(3), pp. 433–442. doi: https://doi.org/10.1016/j.bpg.2013.07.002

Peebles, K.A. and Price, T.J. (2011). Self-injurious behaviour in intellectual disability syndromes: Evidence for aberrant pain signalling as a contributing factor. *Journal of Intellectual Disability Research*, 56(5), pp. 441–452. doi: https://doi.org/10.1111/j.1365-2788.2011.01484.x [Accessed 05.09.2023]

Pouard, T. (2023). Constipation in people with learning disabilities: Prevalence and impact. *Nursing Times*, 119(4), pp. 18–20. Available at: https://search.ebscohost.com/login.aspx?direct=true&db=cul&AN=163129835 [Accessed: 13/02/2024].

Pratt, N.L., Kalisch Ellett, L.M., Sluggett, J.K., Gadzhanova, S.V., Ramsay, E.N., Kerr, M., LeBlanc, V.T., Barratt, J.D. and Roughead, E.E. (2016). Use of proton pump inhibitors among older Australians: National quality improvement programmes have led to sustained practice change. *International Journal for Quality in Health Care*, 29(1), pp. 75–82. doi: https://doi.org/10.1093/intqhc/mzw138

Public Health England (2016). Constipation: Making reasonable adjustments. Available at: https://www.gov.uk/government/publications/constipation-and-people-with-learning-disabilities/constipation-making-reasonable-adjustments [Accessed 14/09/2023]

Purple All Stars (2019). Check me for sepsis. Hertfordshire County Council. *You Tube*. 17 May. Available at: https://www.youtube.com/watch?v=FZq5sYulOB8 [Accessed 09/02/2024]

Regnard, C., Reynolds, J., Watson, B., Matthews, D., Gibson, L. and Clarke, C. (2007). Understanding distress in people with severe communication difficulties: Developing and assessing the Disability Distress Assessment Tool (DisDAT). *Journal of Intellectual Disability Research*, [online] 51(4), pp. 277–292. doi: https://doi.org/10.1111/j.1365-2788.2006.00875 [Accessed 16.10.2023]

Robertson, J., Baines, S., Emerson, E. and Hatton, C. (2018). Prevalence of constipation in people with intellectual disability: A systematic review. *Journal of Intellectual & Developmental Disability*, 43(4), pp. 392–406. doi: https://doi.org/10.3109/13668250.2017.1310829

Ronkainen, J. and Agréus, L. (2013). Epidemiology of reflux symptoms and GORD. *Best Practice & Research Clinical Gastroenterology*, 27(3), pp. 325–337. doi: https://doi.org/10.1016/j.bpg.2013.06.008

Royal College of Nursing. (2021). *Diagnostic overshadowing | Congress Royal College of Nursing*. [online] Available at: https://www.rcn.org.uk/congress/congress-events/diagnostic-overshadowing#:~:text=Diagnostic%20overshadowing%20occurs%20when%20a [Accessed 26.09.2023]

Sanna, L., Stuart, A.L., Berk, M., Pasco, J.A., Girardi, P. and Williams, L.J. (2013). Gastro oesophageal reflux disease (GORD)-related symptoms and its association with mood and anxiety disorders and psychological symptomology: A population-based study in women. *BMC Psychiatry*, 13(1). doi: https://doi.org/10.1186/1471-244x-13-194

Schneider, H. (2007). Gastro-oesophageal reflux disease: The Montreal definition and classification. *South African Family Practice*, 49(1), pp. 19–26. doi: https://doi.org/10.1080/207862 04.2007.10873501

Sherwood Forest Hospitals (2019). Sepsis information for paid carers/professionals of people with a Learning Disability: You Tube. 21 March. Available at: https://www.youtube. com/watch?v=KPY6tLgmChE [Accessed 9/02/2024]

Simpson, N., Mizen, L. and Cooper, S.-A. (2020). Intellectual disabilities. *Medicine*, 48(11). doi: https://doi.org/10.1016/j.mpmed.2020.08.010

Taggart, L., Mulhall, P., Kelly, R., Trip, H., Sullivan, B., and Flygare Wallen, E. (2022). Preventing, mitigating, and managing future pandemics for people with an intellectual and developmental disability- Learnings from COVID-19: A scoping review. *Journal of Policy and Practice in Intellectual Disabilities*, 19(1), pp. 4–34. doi: https://doi.org/10.1111/ jppi.12408

The Caroline Walker Trust (2007). Eating well: Children and adults with learning disabilities Nutritional and practical guidelines (online). Available at: https://www.cwt.org.uk/wp-content/uploads/2015/02/EWLDGuidelines.pdf [Accessed 16.10.2023]

The National Archives (2023). Equality act 2010. [online] Legislation.gov.uk. Available at: https://www.legislation.gov.uk/ukpga/2010/15/contents [Accessed 26.09.2023]

The UK Sepsis Trust (n.d.) A Guide for Patients and Relatives. Available at: https://sepsistrust. org/get-support/support/resources/ [Accessed 09/02/2024]

van Schrojenstein Lantman-de Valk, H.M.J. and Walsh, P.N. (2008). Managing health problems in people with intellectual disabilities. *BMJ*, 337(dec08 1), pp. a2507–a2507. doi: https://doi.org/10.1136/bmj.a2507 [Accessed 05.09.2023]

Wake, A., Davies, J., Drake, C., Rowbotham, M., Smith, N. and Rossiter, R. (2020). Keep Safe: Collaborative practice development and research with people with learning disabilities. *Tizard Learning Disability Review*, 25(4), pp. 173–180. doi: https://doi.org/10.1108/ tldr-12-2019-0040

World Health Organization (2017). Seventieth World Health Assembly Update. Available at: https://leder.nhs.uk/images/annual_reports/leder_annual_report_2016_2017.pdf

World Health Organization (2023). Sepsis Key facts. Available at: https://www.who.int/news-room/fact-sheets/detail/sepsis [Accessed 24/11/2023]

Zhong, X., Ashira-Oredope, D., Pate, A., Martin, G., Sharma, A., Dark, P., Felton, T., Lake, C., Mackenna, B., Mehrkar, A., Bacon, S., Masset, J., Inglesby, P., Goldacre, B., The Open SAFELY Collaborative., Hand, K., Bladon, S., Cunningham, N., Gilham, E., Brown, C., Mirfenderesky, M., Palin, V.and Pieter van Staa, T. (2023). Clinical and health inequality risk factors for non-Covid related sepsis during the global Covid-19 pandemic: a national case control and cohort study. *eClinical medicine*, 23 November, 102321. https://doi.org/10.1016/j.eclinm.2023.102321 [Accessed 24/11/2023]

15

Epilepsy and individuals with a learning disability

Helen Jones

NICE (2022) state that 'Learning disabilities are common in people with epilepsy'. This is an interesting way of phrasing that epilepsy is more common in those who have a learning disability. NICE goes on to outline that it is important that those professionals working with people with epilepsy have an understanding and recognition of the needs of people with a learning disability and that they are able to offer the right support and same level of treatment as those who do not have a learning disability. There have been significant clinical and therapeutic developments over the last century for people with epilepsy but in spite of this they often continue to suffer from discrimination. This can be particularly challenging when those people also have a learning disability.

What NICE and others need to do is to recognise in their research and guidance the importance of understanding the limitations that having epilepsy places on an individual with epilepsy in terms of lifestyle and quality of life (Espie and Kerr, 2013). Due to the high prevalence of epilepsy in people with a learning disability it is important to realise the far-reaching impact meaning that treatment and management needs to reach beyond simply controlling the immediate effect of seizures. Epilepsy for someone with a learning disability is yet another example of co-morbidity which can affect relationships, community participation, activities of daily living as well as its effect on choice, social stigma, behaviour and life expectancy (Robertson et al., 2015). This is significant with prevalence rates being estimated at around 22% compared to around 0.6% of the rest of the population (Robertson et al., 2015). This prevalence rate increases with the severity of learning disability.

This chapter will set out some of the ways in which epilepsy can be considered and therefore supported in a more person-centred way for those who also have a diagnosis of a learning disability. It is not aimed at providing in-depth discussion around protocols, treatment approaches and diagnostic pathways. However, it will consider some of the key recommendations from NICE (2022) alongside some of the more evidence-based approaches to communication and supporting those with a learning disability.

DOI: 10.4324/9781003341765-17

Epilepsy and the myth

As we (society, healthcare professionals, academics and people with epilepsy) have begun to understand epilepsy more over recent years and decades it has become apparent that something so complex and individual to the person means we often misunderstand what we are experiencing and seeing. Advances in neuro-imaging as well as the adoption of the biopsychosocial model of healthcare means that we understand the nature of seizures far more than we did even ten or twenty years ago. The way that seizures are classified has significantly changed (see Figure 15.1) presenting us with different information. Before we begin to consider epilepsy and the care approaches we need to adopt for those with a learning disability we need to understand a little bit more about what we understand and mean by epilepsy. It is important that we dispel any common misunderstanding and myth. The history of epilepsy is entrenched in cultural belief, religious ideology and, crucially, fear! The idea of someone with epilepsy across different times and cultural groups has ranged from the person being held up as divine to demonic (Devinsky and Lai, 2008) and the history of epilepsy is fraught with stigma and at times even persecution (ILAE, 2003)

What is epilepsy?

First of all, think epilepsies rather than epilepsy. Essentially epilepsies are a group of neurological conditions characterised by recurrent seizures. The important word there is the word 'recurrent'. Epilepsy could also be characterised as a physical condition due to its clinical presentation and the effects upon a person's body.

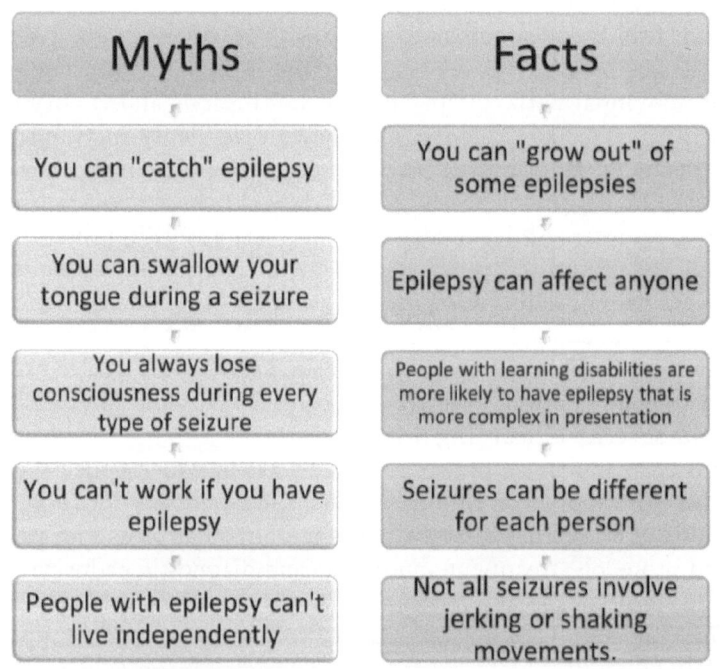

FIGURE 15.1 Myths and facts image design by Matt Kelly

Anyone can have a seizure for many reasons at different stages of their lives but they are not necessarily due to epilepsy. For example, a young infant may have a seizure known commonly as a febrile convulsion due to a spike in temperature but not due to the condition of epilepsy.

Figure 15.2 shows a list of seizure types defined by the International League of Epilepsy in 2017. These are broadly split into generalised (involving both sides of the brain and occurring without warning) and focal onset (involving one part of the brain). Understanding more than how a seizure looks and presents can also support with response, assessment and then treatment approach which is important when caring for someone with a learning disability.

Seizures are now divided into groups depending on:

■   where they start in the brain (onset)

■   whether or not a person's awareness is affected

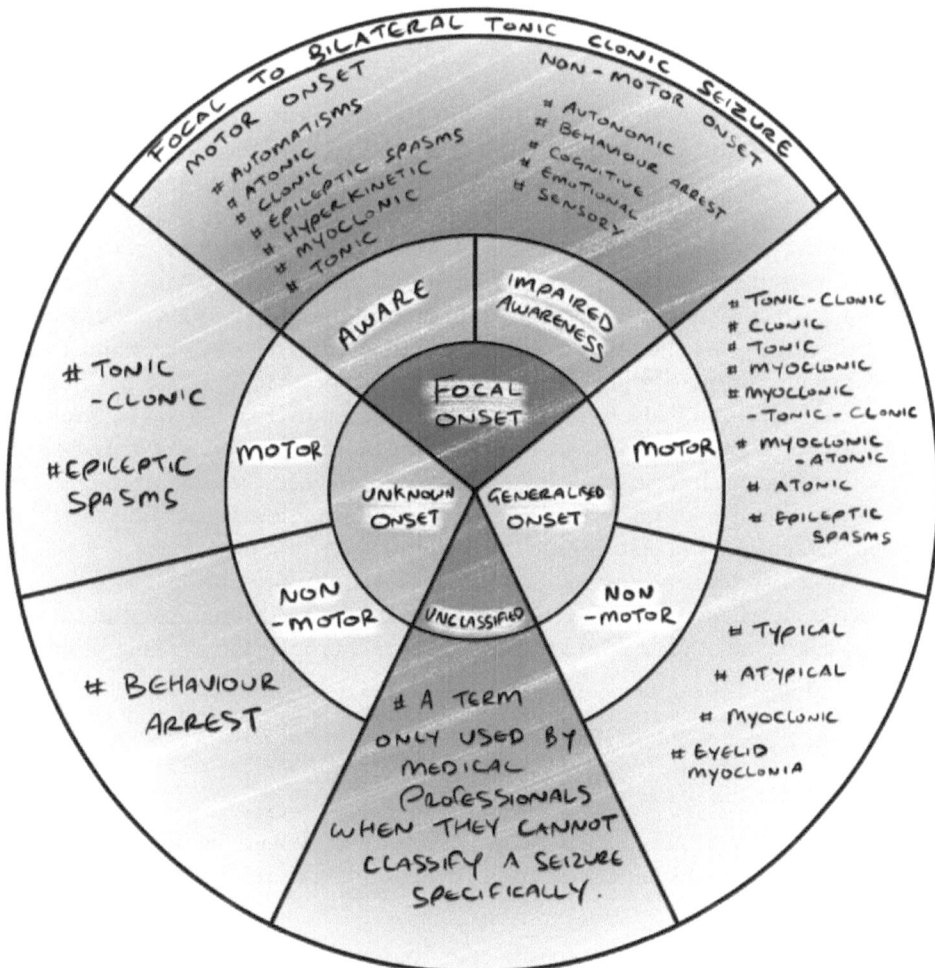

FIGURE 15.2 Seizure classification image design by Matt Kelly

- whether or not seizures involve other symptoms, such as movement
- Depending on where they start, seizures are described as being focal onset, generalised onset or unknown onset.

Seizure types and diagnosis

As the care and treatment of epilepsy has progressed, new discoveries have been made in relation to what we know neurologically about different seizure types. Some of the more commonly known seizure types include tonic-clonic, clonic, atonic, absence and myoclonic seizures (see Figure 15.2). Previously some of these seizure types were referred to in other terms, such as 'petit mal' and 'grand mal' which then developed into terms such as 'complex partial' or 'simple partial'. However, these terms are no longer in use. It is much more important to understand what we actually know, experience and see of a seizure as well as any other associated syndromic diagnosis, aetiology and any other impairments that the individual may have, including that of a learning disability rather than simply stating a seizure type. Consideration of all these aspects together helps us to understand more about a person's epilepsy. This chapter will not explore different seizure types in further detail as it is quite easy to look this information up through different other sources (see 'Useful Links' at the end of the chapter).

One key skill that this chapter will aim to develop and support is the ability to take and record an accurate seizure description. As you can see from Figure 15.2 there are times when the cause of seizures is unknown and it is not uncommon for seizure activity not to be picked up through neurological investigation (Höller et al., 2017). One of the advantages to understanding someone's seizure activity and their epilepsy is when we are able to elicit a comprehensive, clear and accurate seizure description. Simply stating the seizure type that someone has likely experienced (e.g. 'John had a tonic-clonic seizure at 3 p.m. that lasted about ten minutes') is a poor description of a seizure. The reason for this is that we are not provided with sufficient information. In addition to this, when those witnessing a seizure try to describe it without recording all of the information at the time there can often be discrepancies in features such as timing.

When recording a seizure description, we do not need to be too concerned about recording whether this is a generalised atonic seizure, for example. Instead we should describe some of what is listed below that would provide far more useful information:

- What was happening beforehand? How was the person and what were they doing?
- What time of day did this happen?
- Did the person report any changes in how they were feeling or what they were experiencing such as changes in body temperature, feelings of confusion, sensory changes?
- Did the person appear to lose consciousness? (This can be checked through the seizure activity by continually trying to speak to the person.)

- Did you notice any other physical changes? This might include loss of bladder or bowel control, eye rolling or any other movement not usual to the person.

- Were there any changes in behaviour immediately before, during or after the seizure activity?

- Did the person make any sound? Was there a shout, scream, mumbling?

- Did the seizure activity involve movement of any limbs? This may include twitching, jerking movements. If there was which limbs and which side of the body was this?

- How long did the whole seizure activity seem to last for? This should include from the very first small change to the point at which the person appears to be back to their usual self. This should be accurately timed.

All of this information provides a lot of detail and gives indications as to where in the brain a seizure may be occurring, any changes to the person's epilepsy that may need further investigation as well as indicating whether the seizure was generalised or focal onset.

Management of epilepsy and people with learning disabilities

The NICE (2022) guidance on 'Epilepsies in children, young people and adults' reminds us that the best approach to supporting those with learning disabilities and co-morbidities is to be coordinated, to be multi-disciplinary in approach and, most importantly, individualised. This acknowledges the need for individual care planning and coordination including the development of emergency management plans and protocols. NICE guidance supports the access to a specialist epilepsy nurse as a point of contact, education and support. The epilepsy nurse can ensure that the holistic approach to epilepsy care and management is central to the support and guidance given to individuals and their families during assessment, treatment discussions and management over time.

Key areas of support to enable people to self-manage and make informed choices about their own care include:

- Identifying and supporting around potential triggers that may provoke seizures

- Medication and adherence to medication including possible side-effects

- Reducing risks including any risk to SUDEP (sudden unexpected death in epilepsy)

- Lifestyle and activities of daily living

- Associated syndromes and seizure types

It is important that we can identify not only the correct seizure type but its clinical association to any electro-clinical syndrome in order to provide the right diagnostic and treatment pathway for someone with epilepsy. (See 'Useful Links' for further information at the end of the chapter.)

> **TOP TIP**
>
> Use the principles of the Mental Capacity Act (2005) at all times to ensure that a person is empowered to make their own decisions wherever possible about their epilepsy care and to be able to communicate their wishes, feelings and preferences around the way in which their epilepsy is supported and managed. Easy-read and accessible information is important to consider when providing someone with information about their epilepsy.

Associated electroclinical syndromes and learning disabilities

Electroclinical syndromes are epilepsies usually diagnosed in childhood and characterised according age of onset, seizure type, EEG patterns, aetiology and any other associated features. In many cases this may also include a level of learning disability. Knowing whether someone's epilepsy is part of a syndrome is important because it helps us to understand appropriate treatment as well as outcomes and prognosis. Electroclinical syndromes, which move beyond simply providing descriptions of seizure types and frequency of seizure activity, mean that we can more easily take a holistic and evidence-based approach to someone's epilepsy care. Some of the electroclinical syndromes that are more commonly associated with children with a learning disability include:

- Dravet Syndrome
- West Syndrome
- Otahara Syndrome (rare)
- Lennox–Gastaut Syndrome
- Landau Kleffner Syndrome

These are just a few of the electroclinical syndromes associated with epilepsy and a learning disability. It is important that if you are aware of an associated syndrome when supporting someone who has epilepsy that you are able to find out as much as you can about the condition, its prevalence and the way in which it can be managed (see 'Useful Links' at the end of the chapter). Family and person-centred approaches mean that often nurses and other health professionals are the key people involved in education and signposting around support and understanding. It is important that hospital appointments are made accessible using tools such as hospital passports and other appropriate communication methods for that individual. Epilepsy is a frightening and sometimes life-threatening condition which families will need guidance and support with. In addition to this the risks associated with epileptic seizures mean that often individuals may find their quality of life and access to certain opportunities more limited and this along with suitable treatment and medication regimes needs to be carefully considered.

Lifestyle and risk management

Within other areas of healthcare, including mental health and risk management, particular approaches and processes support with ensuring that a person is not managed in overly restrictive manner. Principle 5 as outlined by the Mental Capacity Act (2005) relates specifically to any decision being made in a person's best interests as needing to be always the least restrictive option and that we should take into account the wishes of the person themselves. One model of risk management that has been embraced by professionals working within learning disability specialist services for many years is the positive risk management approach developed and endorsed by Steve Morgan. Morgan (2010) analyses this approach as emerging predominantly from a forensic base and being responsive to an ever increasing social demand on containing risk and ensuring there is accountability. Steve Morgan states that 'trying to remove risk from anyone's life is tantamount to depriving them of an essential element that contributes to quality of life – we all need to take risks to reap the benefits of our chosen endeavours' (Morgan, 2010, p. 20). Positive risk-taking as outlined by Morgan is characterised by weighing up benefits with potential harms and ensuring that all priorities of the individual themselves are also considered within this process and any subsequent actions and planning.

What has this all to do with epilepsy? The principles of positive risk-taking can be well applied to management of this condition with individuals who also have a learning disability. Having a learning disability can be hugely restrictive anyway in terms of choice, life experience, health outcomes and this can relate to areas including employment, education and relationships. Epilepsy is also a restrictive condition within society. There are choices to be made around treatment that may cause significant side effects. There may be associated risk with carrying out daily living tasks such as travelling alone, having a bath alone and even taking part in certain extra-curricular activities such as swimming or socialising with friends. It is important that to enhance and maximise someone's quality of life their wishes and strengths are considered, that nurses and other health professionals build trusting relationships so that any information about their epilepsy is communicated in a way to enable them to be involved in planning their own care and making informed decisions.

TOP TIP

Consider how positive risk taking can be built into care planning and person-centred planning. Try to capture the wishes and thoughts of the individual and to present these wherever possible to those responsible for overseeing the treatment and management of the person's epilepsy. If you are responsible for overseeing and managing, consider how elements such as staffing and training can support this approach.

This chapter has highlighted the way in which we now classify and understand someone's epilepsy based on a holistic, positive risk-taking approach. The role of the nurse or other health professionals has been highlighted in the role they can play in supporting diagnosis and communication for the person and their families as well as being introduced to the idea of understanding the epilepsies from a syndromic diagnosis and treatment perspective.

Useful links

Epilepsy Society: https://epilepsysociety.org.uk/about-epilepsy/epileptic-seizures/seizure-types

https://epilepsysociety.org.uk/blog/ilae-new-seizure-classification

ILEA (International League Against Epilepsy): https://www.ilae.org/guidelines/definition-and-classification/classification-and-definition-of-epilepsy-syndromes

References

Devinsky, O. and Lai, G. (2008) Spirituality and religion in epilepsy. *Epilepsy & Behavior, 12*(4), 636–643.

Espie, C.A. and Kerr, M. (2013) 'Epilepsy and learning disability: Implications for quality of life'. In *Quality of Life in Epilepsy* (pp. 145–158). Psychology Press.

Höller, Y., Uhl, A., Bathke, A., Thomschewski, A., Butz, K., Nardone, R., Fell, J. and Trinka, E. (2017) Reliability of EEG measures of interaction: a paradigm shift is needed to fight the reproducibility crisis. *Frontiers in Human Neuroscience, 11*, 441.

ILAE (2003) The history and stigma of epilepsy. *Epilepsia*, 44: 1214. https://doi.org/10.1046/j.1528-1157.44.s.6.2.x

Morgan, S. (2010) Positive risk taking: a basis for good risk decision-making. *Health Care Risk Report, 16*(4), 20–21.

National Institute for Health and Care Excellence (NICE) (2022) Epilepsies in children, young people and adults NG217. https://www.nice.org.uk/guidance/ng217 (Accessed on 24.04.2023)

Robertson, J., Hatton, C., Emerson, E. and Baines, S., (2015) Prevalence of epilepsy among people with intellectual disabilities: a systematic review. *Seizure, 29*, 46–62.

16

Learning disabilities and stroke

Sarah Davies

Introduction to stroke within a learning disability context

Stroke, a common and complex neurovascular disease, is a major cause of mortality and morbidity (Williams et al., 2019). Principally there are two types of stroke. Ischemic strokes account for the majority of cases and occur due to clots or blockages of blood vessels leading to the brain. Haemorrhagic strokes are due to a ruptured artery increasing pressure in cells, resulting in brain damage (Centre for Disease Control and Prevention, 2023). Transient ischemic attacks are sometimes referred to as 'mini-strokes'; they can be predictive of future strokes, characterised by sudden cognitive deficits that resolve within 24 hours (National Institute for Health and Care Excellence [NICE], 2023a).

Stroke results in neurological deficits (Williams et al., 2019). It is important to note that this type of acquired brain injury is different from a learning disability where the onset occurs in childhood (NICE, 2023b). The prevalence of stroke is increased for people with learning disabilities compared with the general population (Cooper et al., 2018) and it is a preventable cause of death for this group (Learning Disability Mortality Review, 2021). Young et al. (2020) suggest that health outcomes following a stroke are poorer for those with learning disabilities and specific medical interventions, such as thrombolysis (administration of alteplase medication to disperse a clot), can be withheld; this inequality may be due to limited research or complex ethical considerations.

Health inequalities: how does this relate to stroke?

Health inequalities are widely documented in disadvantaged groups and those living with disability (The King's Fund, 2023). Almost 50% of individuals with a learning disability are thought to die due to avoidable causes of death; with cardiovascular disease being a leading reason (Learning Disability Mortality Review [LeDeR], 2021). Sedentary behaviour, obesity and an unhealthy lifestyle are

DOI: 10.4324/9781003341765-18

modifiable contributors to stroke, these areas should be actively addressed as they are of increasing concern for individuals with a learning disability (LeDeR, 2019; Lynch et al., 2022).

Detection of stroke: why might stroke be harder to recognise in people with learning disabilities?

The FAST (face, arms, speech time) test; whereby facial droop, unilateral arm weakness or movement and slurred or garbled speech indicates time critical medical intervention is needed for the initiation of assessment and treatment of a potential stroke (Stroke Guideline, 2023). This screening tool used by clinicians is the focus of mass media campaigns improving public awareness of stroke.

The **F**acial features of people with learning disabilities can be distinctive and vary in comparison with the general population. They are often associated with genetic disorders including Down syndrome (Centers for Disease Control and Prevention, 2024). This may result in facial changes due to stroke onset not being recognised among people with learning disabilities especially as medical professionals often have limited awareness and understanding of learning disabilities (NHS England and NHS Improvement, 2019).

Some people with learning disabilities may have weakened limbs or unusual/involuntary movements of **A**rms; therefore observable weakening of arms may not be applicable or go unrecognised as a symptom of stroke.

As previously noted changes in **S**peech can be indicative of stroke onset; however, speech, language and communication needs and abilities of people with learning disabilities are wide ranging and often overlooked (Royal College of Speech and Language Therapists, 2023) meaning potential further difficulties in recognition and diagnosis of stroke.

Diagnostic overshadowing (whereby symptoms occurring from ill health are attributed to the learning disability) (NHS England, 2023a) is another consideration for stroke recognition in this patient group. Behaviour changes and symptoms that occur due to stroke may differ in comparison with the general population or be misattributed to learning disability (NHS England, 2023a); furthermore, there may be a lack of help seeking behaviour (e.g. pain and physiological sensations may not be communicated or there may be a delay in alerting others to the need for intervention). There is increased likelihood of epilepsy and seizure activity within the learning disability population which can occur as part of a stroke, however they are also considered 'stroke mimics' (Mangiardi et al., 2021) hence this could create obscured assessment and **T**imely intervention.

Support needs are likely to change with age and in the occurrence of stroke; an end-of-life care plan is an important consideration (NICE, 2018). Care must be tailored to the individual and be person-centred, involve speech and language therapists and dietitians if needed. Involvement of appropriate family members and/or advocates is essential.

Spring 2024 saw the launch of a digital cardiovascular health check. This could improve stroke prevention by indicating the need for statins to reduce cholesterol enabling patients to be reviewed by their GP (Department of Health and Social Care, 2023). However it would be important to evaluate the efficacy of this new technology, especially in relation to people with learning disabilities.

What care is needed for people with learning disabilities following a stroke?

The National Stroke Service Model (2021) details best practice for care and treatment of stroke patients; therefore key considerations related to learning disabilities are discussed below.

Prevention strategies: along with joint decision making, the importance of communication and involvement of family and carers is highlighted, along with the importance of health checks and health action plans.

Pre-hospital care aims to screen and triage so treatment is not delayed. Immediate transfer to hospital should be arranged and achieved within a 180-minute timeframe. Although admission to hospital may be unplanned in the event of stroke, anticipatory measures should be taken to prepare individuals in the event of an emergency (The Regulation and Quality Improvement Authority, 2018). This may involve completing/updating a person's hospital passport and supporting them to pack an emergency overnight bag (NHS, 2022b) as well as discussing hospital care, using easy-read guides can prove to be a useful tool (Social Care Institute for Excellence, n.d.).

The **hyperacute phase** is considered to take place in the first 72 hours after admission; patients should be cared for by a specialist stroke team and receive input from the MDT (e.g. learning disability hospital liaison nurse, physiotherapist, speech and language therapist, occupational therapist and dietitian). Neurovascular imaging should inform diagnosis and management (e.g. IV thrombolysis). A swallow screen to indicate the presence of dysphasia is a priority to reduce risk of stroke-related pneumonia (National Stroke Programme Working Group – Swallow Screen Sub-Group, 2017). Continuous specialist care should take place in the **acute treatment phase** when a venous thromboembolism (VTE) risk assessment should take place and intermittent pneumatic compression should be prescribed if appropriate reducing the risk of blood clots developing (NICE, 2019). Inpatient rehabilitation should also commence along with appropriate protocols to prevent pressure ulcers (e.g. repositioning regimes) (NICE, 2014) and manage bladder and bowel continence (urinary catheterisation should be avoided if possible) (NICE, 2023c).

Rehabilitation focuses on improving quality of life for those affected by stroke and achieving goals based on individual needs. The Integrated Community Stroke Service aims to ensure patient goals are set and reviewed to achieve measurable benefit; frequency and duration of rehabilitation input should be based on individual need. When appropriate the management plan should be shared with carers and their needs assessed.

Further resources

Health Education England (2021): https://www.hee.nhs.uk/sites/default/files/documents/Stroke%20Training%20Guide.pdf

HSE: https://www.hse.ie/eng/about/who/cspd/ncps/stroke/resources/national-clinical-guideline-for-stroke.pdf

Mencap (2023): https://www.mencap.org.uk/advice-and-support/health-coronavirus/health-guides

NHS England (2017): https://www.england.nhs.uk/wp-content/uploads/2017/05/nat-elec-health-check-ld-clinical-template.pdf

NHS Derbyshire Healthcare (2023): https://www.derbyshirehealthcareft.nhs.uk/services/learning-disabilities/annual-health-check/7-health-action-plan

NHS (2021): https://www.england.nhs.uk/wp-content/uploads/2021/05/stroke-service-model-may-2021.pdf

NICE (2022): https://www.nice.org.uk/guidance/ng128/resources/stroke-and-transient-ischaemic-attack-in-over-16s-diagnosis-and-initial-management-pdf-66141665603269

References

Centers for Disease Control and Prevention (2024) About Stroke. Available at: [Accessed 02.01.2024]. https://www.cdc.gov/birth-defects/about/down-syndrome.html

Cooper, S. et al. (2018) Management and prevalence of long-term conditions in primary health care for adults with intellectual disabilities compared with the general population: a population-based cohort study. *Journal of Applied Research in Intellectual Disabilities*, 31 (S1), 68–81. Available at: https://onlinelibrary-wiley-com.bcu.idm.oclc.org/doi/pdf/10.1111/jar.12386 [Accessed 02.01.2024].

Department for Health and Social Care (2023) New digital health check to tackle deadly cardiovascular disease. Available at: https://www.gov.uk/government/news/new-digital-health-check-to-tackle-deadly-cardiovascular-disease [Accessed 04.01.02024].

Learning Disability Mortality Review (2019) Learning Disabilities Mortality Review (LeDeR) Programme: Fact Sheet 28. Available at: https://www.bristol.ac.uk/media-library/sites/sps/leder/2103_Nutrition_PDF.pdf [Accessed 04.01.2024].

Learning Disability Mortality Review (2021) Action from Learning Report 2020/21. Available at: https://www.england.nhs.uk/wp-content/uploads/2021/06/LeDeR-Action-from-learning-report-202021.pdf [Accessed 04.01.2024].

Learning Disability Mortality Review (2021) Action from Learning Report 2020/2021. Available at: https://www.england.nhs.uk/wp-content/uploads/2021/06/LeDeR-Action-from-learning-report-202021.pdf [Accessed 02.01.2024].

Lynch, L. et al. (2022) Physical health effects of sedentary behaviour on adults with an intellectual disability: a scoping review. *Journal of Intellectual Disabilities*. https://doi.org/10.1177/17446295221107281

Mangiardi, M., Anticoli, S., Bertaccini, L., Cozzolino, V. & Pezzella, F. R. (2021) Acute Onset Focal Epilepsy Mimicking Stroke. *Cureus*, 13(10), e18600. https://doi.org/10.7759/cureus.18600

National Institute for Health and Care Excellence (2014) Pressure ulcers: prevention and management. Available at: https://www.nice.org.uk/guidance/cg179/resources/pressure-ulcers-prevention-and-management-pdf-35109760631749 [Accessed 03.01.2024].

National Institute for Health and Care Excellence (2016) Mental health problems in people with learning disabilities: prevention, assessment and management. Available at: https://www.nice.org.uk/guidance/ng54/resources/mental-health-problems-in-people-with-learning-disabilities-prevention-assessment-and-management-pdf-1837513295557 [Accessed 03.01.2024].

National Institute for Health and Care Excellence (2018) Care and support of people growing older with learning disabilities. Available at: https://www.nice.org.uk/guidance/ng96/resources/care-and-support-of-people-growing-older-with-learning-disabilities-pdf-1837758519493 [accessed 02.01.2024].

National Institute for Health and Care Excellence (2019) Venous thromboembolism in over 16s: reducing the risk of hospital-acquired deep vein thrombosis or pulmonary embolism. Available at: https://www.nice.org.uk/guidance/ng89/resources/venous-thromboembolism-in-over-16s-reducing-the-risk-of-hospitalacquired-deep-vein-thrombosis-or-pulmonary-embolism-pdf-1837703092165 [Accessed 02.01.2024].

National Institute for Health and Care Excellence (2022) Stroke and transient ischaemic attack in over 16s: diagnosis and initial management. Available at: https://www.nice.org.uk/guidance/ng128/resources/stroke-and-transient-ischaemic-attack-in-over-16s-diagnosis-and-initial-management-pdf-66141665603269 [Accessed 02.01.2024].

National Institute for Health and Care Excellence (2023a) What are the clinical features of stroke and TIA? Available at: https://cks.nice.org.uk/topics/stroke-tia/diagnosis/clinical-features/ [Accessed 02.01.2024].

National Institute for Health and Care Excellence (2023b) Learning Disabilities: What is it? Available at: https://cks.nice.org.uk/topics/learning-disabilities/background-information/definition/ [Accessed 02.01.2024].

National Institute for Health and Care Excellence (2023c) Urinary incontinence in neurological disease: assessment and management. Available at: https://www.nice.org.uk/guidance/cg148/resources/urinary-incontinence-in-neurological-disease-assessment-and-management-pdf-35109577553605 [Accessed 02.01.2024].

National Institute of Neurological Disorders and Stroke (2023c) Sotos Syndrome. Available at: https://www.ninds.nih.gov/health-information/disorders/sotos-syndrome [Accessed 02.01.2024].

National Institute of Neurological Disorders and Stroke (2023e) NICE Impact People with a Learning disability. Available at: https://www.nice.org.uk/about/what-we-do/into-practice/measuring-the-use-of-nice-guidance/impact-of-our-guidance/nice-impact-people-with-a-learning-disability [Accessed 04.01.2024].

National Stroke Programme Working Group – Swallow Screen Sub-Group (2017) National Guideline for Swallow Screening in Stroke 2017. Available at: https://www.hse.ie/eng/services/publications/clinical-strategy-and-programmes/national-guideline-for-swallow-screening-in-stroke-hse.pdf [Accessed 03.01.2024].

NHS (2017) Stroke Services: Configuration Decision Support Guide Appendices. Available at: https://www.england.nhs.uk/mids-east/wp-content/uploads/sites/7/2017/07/configuration-decision-support-guide-appendices-2.pdf [Accessed 04.05.2024].

NHS (2019) The NHS Long Term Plan. Available at: https://www.longtermplan.nhs.uk/wp-content/uploads/2019/01/nhs-long-term-plan-june-2019.pdf [Accessed 03.01.2024].

NHS (2022a) Annual Health Checks. Available at: https://www.nhs.uk/conditions/learning-disabilities/annual-health-checks/ [Accessed 02.01.2024].

NHS (2022b) Support if you are going into hospital. Available at: https://www.nhs.uk/conditions/learning-disabilities/going-into-hospital/ [Accessed 02.01.2024].

NHS England (2018) Guide to making information accessible for people with a learning disability. Available at: https://www.england.nhs.uk/wp-content/uploads/2018/06/LearningDisabilityAccessCommsGuidance.pdf [Accessed 04.01.2024].

NHS England (2023a) Clinical guide for front line staff to support the management of patients with a learning disability and autistic people – relevant to all clinical specialties. Available at: https://www.england.nhs.uk/long-read/clinical-guide-for-front-line-staff-to-support-the-management-of-patients-with-a-learning-disability-and-autistic-people-relevant-to-all-clinical-specialties/ [Accessed 03.01.2024].

NHS England (2023b) Why is it important to involve people. Available at: https://www.england.nhs.uk/learning-disabilities/about/get-involved/involving-people/why-is-it-important-to-involve-people/ [Accessed 02.01.2024].

NHS England (2024) *Improving Health*. Available at: https://www.england.nhs.uk/learning-disabilities/improving-health/ [Accessed 22.01.24].

NHS England and NHS Improvement. (2019) Learning Disability Mortality Review (LeDeR) Programme: Action from Learning. Nation Health Service England. Available at: https://www.england.nhs.uk/wp-content/uploads/2019/05/action-from-learning.pdf [Accessed 02.01.2024].

NHS Health Education England (2023) The Oliver McGowan Mandatory Training on Learning Disability and Autism. Available at: https://www.hee.nhs.uk/our-work/learning-disability/current-projects/oliver-mcgowan-mandatory-training-learning-disability-autism#:~:text=The%20Health%20and%20Care%20Act,training%20appropriate%20to%20their%20role [Accessed 02.01.2024].

Public Health England (2016) Annual health checks and people with learning disabilities. Available at: https://www.gov.uk/government/publications/annual-health-checks-and-people-with-learning-disabilities/annual-health-checks-and-people-with-learning-disabilities [Accessed 02.01.2024].

Public Health England (2017) Improving the Health and Wellbeing of People with Learning Disabilities. Available at: https://assets.publishing.service.gov.uk/media/5a8211c6ed915d74e34018f2/Health_charter_2017_guidance.pdf [Accessed 02.01.2024].

Public Health England (2018) Briefing document: First incidence of stroke Estimates for England 2007 to 2016. Available at: https://assets.publishing.service.gov.uk/media/5a82ab52e5274a2e8ab58bb5/Stroke_incidence_briefing_document_2018.pdf [Accessed 03.01.2024].

Public Health England (2021) Guide to the cardiovascular disease (CVD) prevention programme supporting data packs. Available at: https://fingertips.phe.org.uk/profile/cardiovascular-disease-prevention [Accessed 02.01.2024].

Public Health England (2023) Learning Disabilities – Applying all our Health. Available at: https://www.gov.uk/government/publications/learning-disability-applying-all-our-health/learning-disabilities-applying-all-our-health [Accessed 04.01.2024].

Royal College of Speech and Language Therapists (2023) Learning Disabilities Overview. Available at: https://www.rcslt.org/speech-and-language-therapy/clinical-information/learning-disabilities/ [Accessed 03.01.2024].

Social Care Institute for Excellence (n.d.) Helping you through a hospital stay: Easy Read. Available at: https://www.scie.org.uk/publications/misc/hospitaldischarge/files/hospitaldischarge-easyread.pdf [Accessed 02.01.2024].

Stroke Guideline (2023) National Clinical Guidance for Stroke [PDF]. Available at: https://www.hse.ie/eng/about/who/cspd/ncps/stroke/resources/national-clinical-guideline-for-stroke.pdf [Accessed 02.01.2024].

The King's Fund (2023) https://www.kingsfund.org.uk/insight-and-analysis/blogs/understanding-experience-disabled-people-england

The Regulation and Quality Improvement Authority (2018) Guidelines on Caring for People with a Learning Disability in General Hospital Settings. Available at: https://www.rqia. org.uk/RQIA/files/41/41a812c6-fee8-45ba-81b8-9ed4106cf49a.pdf [Accessed 02.01.2024].

Williams, J., Perry, L., & Watkins, C. (2019) *Stroke Nursing* (2nd edn). Available at: https:// ebookcentral.proquest.com/lib/bcu/reader.action?docID=5726048 [Accessed 02.01.2024].

Young, M. J. et al. (2020) Disabling stroke in persons already with a disability: Ethical dimensions and directives. *Neurology*, 94 (7), 306–310. Available at: https://europepmc.org/ backend/ptpmcrender.fcgi?accid=PMC7176295&blobtype=pdf [Accessed 02.01.2024].

17

The Mental Capacity Act and consent

Helen Jones

Mental capacity and understanding of this term in relation to the Mental Capacity Act (2005) is always on any current strategic agenda in relation to patient and service user care. What we know in relation to people with a learning disability and other associated health conditions is that healthcare and social care professional knowledge is poor in its appropriate and effective application of the Act (House of Lords Select Committee, 2014). LeDeR annual reports consistently identify Mental Capacity Act knowledge as being an important feature often identified through reviews and in some cases as actively contributing to avoidable death and poor care.

In my previous role as a nurse educator within a university setting, I spent much of my time trying to get students to become enthusiastic about important legal frameworks and how they would apply to their everyday nursing practice. This included the issue of mental capacity and its legal application to nursing practice. I told students that when I was working as a community nurse I had the five principles of the Mental Capacity Act written on a small card and stuck inside of the front page of my work notebook. As nurses and health professionals we are often needing to be task focused, ensuring we can carry out complex procedures competently, or remembering important information relating to medication and the conditions they are being used for. This is of course a fundamental and vital part of nursing practice, but our work is almost meaningless without consideration of a person's wishes, level of understanding, and ability to communicate their needs at the most vulnerable times of their life. The Mental Capacity Act is designed to provide protection and to empower as well as to define the duties that professionals are required to undertake and adhere to. The Mental Capacity Act is not designed to prove someone is not able to consent. This is the position all professionals should take when using the principles of the Mental Capacity Act.

DOI: 10.4324/9781003341765-19

The five principles of the Mental Capacity Act (2005)

The five principles of the Mental Capacity Act are as follows:

1 Always assume the person is able to make the decision until you have proof they are not.

2 Try everything possible to support the person make the decision themselves.

3 Do not assume the person does not have capacity to make a decision just because they make a decision that you think is unwise or wrong.

4 If you make a decision for someone who cannot make it themselves, the decision must always be in their best interests.

5 Any decisions, treatment or care for someone who lacks capacity must always follow the path that is the least restrictive of their basic *rights* and freedoms.

Figure 17.1 helps to clearly identify these principles in terms of how we should consider them and approach them when supporting an individual to make a decision about their lives and their care. The *first three principles* help us to consider the level of understanding someone may have, to always work from the assumption that we should seek to show capacity using every means possible before a decision is

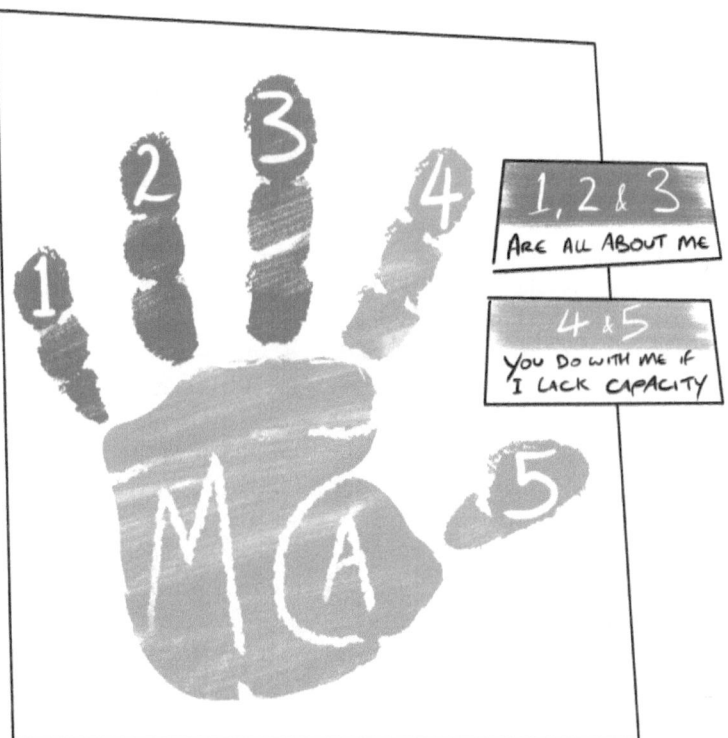

FIGURE 17.1 Principles of MCA design by Matt Kelly

made that someone does not have capacity. The *final two principles* hold us to account as professionals to always ensure that we are doing what is right for that person when they are not able to make a decision about something and that whatever we do is the least restrictive for them.

Always remember: A person may have capacity to make some decisions but not all decisions. Always challenge anyone who makes a sweeping statement of 'they don't have capacity'! Ensure that you are able to ask what decision specifically they are referring to.

When we work with people with learning disabilities we know that putting these principles into practice can be more challenging and we need to become a little more creative to ensure that someone is fully supported to be able to make a decision about their lives or their care. Key things to remember are putting the person at ease, ensuring that appropriate communication is facilitated and that all relevant information is provided in a way that they are more likely to be able to understand (in various chapters easy-read documentation has been discussed and resources recommended that can be used). Underpinning all of this are the key skills associated with nursing and being a healthcare professional including having patience and taking the appropriate amount of time to assess capacity (NMC, 2018). It is really important that you take steps to enable an individual to make their own decisions. It is also important that you have the courage to challenge anyone who does not adhere to the principles of the Act by becoming an advocate for the rights of that individual (DoH, 2012).

Best Interests

How often do we hear 'it was in their best interests' or 'that was done in their best interests'? The term 'Best Interests' as defined within the Mental Capacity Act (2005) has a clear meaning and can only be applied if the person has been shown to lack capacity in relation to a specific decision regarding their care. For a group of health professionals to act in someone's Best Interests they must be able to show that all steps have been taken to support someone to be able to make their own decision in accordance with the *five principles* and the guidance for assessment of mental capacity.

In my experience when undertaking my PhD and in my clinical practice and even as a personal tutor of student nurses and apprentices I came across situations where there was distinct lack of understanding of the term 'Best Interests' and its place within the Mental Capacity Act (2005). The next part of this chapter is setting out what you must consider in your practice when someone *lacks capacity*.

If the person is shown to lack capacity then the following Best Interests checklist must be adhered to. The checklist as defined within the Act is shown on the next page but do remember that what is in someone's Best Interests may change over time and is not fixed. The checklist may also be the starting point but with more complex decisions may need additional considerations or professional involvement. No adult can automatically make a decision on behalf of another adult simply based upon their professional status or personal relationship with the person. A Best Interests decision must be carefully considered as part of a multi-disciplinary approach and this is good practice even when other legal safeguards are in place such as Lasting Power of Attorney (LPA).

- Working out what is in someone's best interests cannot be based simply on someone's age, appearance, condition or behaviour.

- All relevant circumstances should be considered when working out someone's best interests.

- Every effort should be made to encourage and enable the person who lacks capacity to take part in making the decision.

- If there is a chance that the person will regain the capacity to make a particular decision, then it may be possible to put off the decision until later if it is not urgent.

- The person's past and present wishes and feelings, beliefs and values should be taken into account.

- The views of other people who are close to the person who lacks capacity should be considered, as well as the views of an attorney or deputy.

This is all just a reminder really because all of this information can be accessed easily via mandatory training or online resources (see 'Useful Links' at the end of the chapter). The important thing to remember is how to use accessible information, make reasonable adjustments and try to involve the person in the decision-making process. The Act also provides protection for the staff and those caring for an individual. This enables staff to be protected when decisions are made in someone's best interests as well as protecting the rights of the person themselves as long as the steps are followed correctly.

TOP TIP

Use the Code of Practice to the Mental Capacity Act (see 'Useful Links' at the end of the chapter) for practical guidance to using the Act. The Code of Practice contains many scenarios to describe the ways the Act should be used so that it makes more practical sense.

Undertaking a mental capacity test

A common misconception of a mental capacity test is that there is a set, validated tool that can be used for every occasion to assess someone's mental capacity and explore their ability to make an informed decision. A capacity test is based upon a set of guidelines and key statements as set out within the Mental Capacity Act (2005). The way in which it is undertaken should reflect key principles around working with individuals with a learning disability. This means making all reasonable adjustments necessary, adapting communication where needed and ensuring that all information is provided in a way that is accessible for the person. *Remember, the mental capacity test is there to find out whether there is a way to enable capacity and choice*. The person with a learning disability must be over 16 years old and the decision being discussed must relate to the person's health, social care or finances. The capacity test has four parts and failure on any one part indicates a lack of capacity to make the *specific decision* in question at that particular point in time that the decision needs to be made. Time and issues specific is key to the capacity test and assessment of someone's ability to make that decision.

A person is unable to make a decision if they cannot:

1 understand information about the decision to be made (the Act calls this 'relevant information')

2 retain that information in their mind

3 use or weigh that information as part of the decision-making process, or

4 communicate their decision (by talking, using sign language or any other means).

TOP TIP

Think about the people best involved in this assessment process. Think about who knows the person well, understands the way in which they communicate and those who are responsible for proposing the intervention or treatment that the decision is based upon. Remember, the mental capacity test is there to find out whether there is a way to enable capacity and choice.

Advocacy: the role of the Independent Mental Capacity Advocate (IMCA)

Advocacy is an important part of the Mental Capacity Act (2005). It is very important that someone with a learning disability is given the opportunity to have an Independent Mental Capacity Advocate (IMCA) allocated to work with and for them when decisions are being looked at in relation to their health and social care. An IMCA provides support throughout the decision-making process to enable the voice of the person with a learning disability to be heard. They are able to obtain and evaluate relevant information to the person's care including health records and to help ascertain what the person's wishes and beliefs may be and to challenge the decision making process when the principles of best interests need to be adhered to. IMCAs are there to represent the person but also to work alongside the care team as decisions are being explored around healthcare and treatment. The important point to remember is that the IMCA is independent. They do not influence the best interests decision making from a clinical perspective but continue to represent the wishes of the person where appropriate. It is very important that all professionals are aware of the role of the IMCA and its ability to provide vital support to the individual with a learning disability. The House of Lords Post-Legislative Scrutiny Committee on the Mental Capacity Act (2005) reported on 13 March 2014 that the Mental Capacity Act was a good act in principle but that it had to that date been poorly implemented (Bartlett, 2014). Some of the discussion within this report relates to consistency of provision and uptake of the role rather than its value in principle.

> **TOP TIP**
>
> Any Mental Capacity Assessment recording or paperwork within your organisation, provides a checklist which includes a reminder about the IMCA. Make a point of finding out how to contact your local IMCA service and including this information in any relevant policies and documentation relating to capacity assessment.

Advocacy: your role

Within the Code of Practice (NMC, 2018) the importance of acting as an advocate for those in your care is highlighted. Even though the above section stresses the relevance of an IMCA do not underestimate the value and importance of you speaking up for the individual that you are caring for. The IMCA is a defined role as set out by the legal framework of the Mental Capacity Act (2005) but your role as a healthcare professional also requires you to consider how you advocate for those in your care.

> **TOP TIP**
>
> Go back to the NMC Code of Practice or any other Code of Practice that supports you as a healthcare professional and consider the guidance on being a good advocate.

Deprivation of Liberty Safeguards (DoLS)

In 2009, the Deprivation of Liberty Safeguards (DoLS) were included as an amendment to the Mental Capacity Act (2005). They essentially provide the power using the Act to detain a person who lacks capacity if it is felt that is in their best interests. They only apply to adults over 18 years of age. Currently the DoLS criteria only apply to those resident in either a care home or a hospital (the guidance includes all institutions registered as a hospital including mental health). The Deprivation of Liberty Safeguards are due to change to being called the Liberty Protection Safeguards (LPS) and this will also change the criteria against which these can be applied, including the setting. Therefore because the changes have not yet occurred at the time of printing this book please see 'Useful Links' at the end of this chapter for further information.

While DoLS can be used to restrict the care, treatment in a particular environment of someone with a learning disability and essentially deprive them of their liberty in order to ensure that treatment can be offered, there are safeguards in place and DoLS can currently only be authorised under the Court of Protection. The check that needs to be done to consider whether someone who cannot give valid consent to their living arrangements and treatment needs to be legally deprived of their liberty under the Mental Capacity Act is to establish the following:

- Is the person under continuous supervision and control?
- Is the person not free to leave the place where they are living? (This is tested less by what the person says or does but the way staff would react if the person tried to leave.)

If all of the above is true then the person is deprived of their liberty.

Once this check is completed for any informal patients (not legally detained under the Mental Health Act, 1983) then all care and treatment must be reviewed to see if there are any less restrictive ways of providing that care and treatment in accordance with the principles of the Mental Capacity Act. If there are no alternative and less restrictive ways to provide care and treatment then either the Mental Health Act 1983 or the DoLS Safeguards must be considered and implemented. At all times professionals need to show they are working closely with local authority colleagues in implementing the safeguards. All DoLS requests must also be reported to the CQC.

TOP TIP

Find out about the way authorisation for a DoLS is carried out in your area of work. Who is the appropriate supervisory body to advise you within your area? What forms or applications need to be completed? Familiarise yourself with timescales and the difference between a standard authorisation and an urgent authorisation.

It has been mentioned that DoLS will change to LPS. Do keep checking for updates on these changes and familiarise yourself with the differences as well as the similarities.

It can appear that changes occur very quickly after we are only just getting used to what DoLS is and means. However, the LPS has been designed to respond to the feedback from healthcare professionals that DoLS is complex and is therefore not always implemented correctly.

Conclusion and reflection

This chapter has outlined the key principles of the Mental Capacity Act (2005) and provided tips for health and social care professionals so that they are able to understand the importance of using the Act in everyday practice and the ways in which the Act can support people with a learning disability. It is also important in supporting staff and carers to provide the best support to a person keeping in mind important principles such as empowerment, communication and inclusion.

I would like to conclude this chapter by reminding readers about our case studies at the beginning of this book and in particular that of Laura Booth. I would invite you to read this case study again and consider how opportunities to follow the principles of the Act and use Best Interests were missed, ultimately being identified as contributing factors in Laura's death. The Act is there to protect and to empower individuals with a learning disability and their families. We have a legal responsibility to adhere to it at all times and hopefully this chapter can support you to do that in your practice going forward.

Useful links

https://www.scie.org.uk/mca/dols/at-a-glance/#:~:text=The%20Deprivation%20
of%20Liberty%20Safeguards%20(DoLS)%20is%20the%20procedure%20
prescribed,keep%20them%20safe%20from%20harm.

https://www.gov.uk/government/publications/mental-capacity-act-code-of-
practice

References

Bartlett, P. (2014). Good act, poor implementation: the report of the House of Lords Post-Legislative Scrutiny Committee on the Mental Capacity Act 2005. *Elder LJ*, 157.

Department of Health (DoH) (2012). *Compassion in Practice: Nursing, Midwifery and Care Staff – Our Vision and Strategy*. London: Department of Health.

House of Lords Select Committee on the Mental Capacity Act 2005, (2014). Mental Capacity Act 2005: Post-Legislative scrutiny, HL (2013-14) 139. Available online at http://www.parliament.uk/business/committees/committees-a-z/lords-select/mental-capacity-act2005/.) [Accessed on 18/11/2023]

Mental Capacity Act (2005), c. 9. Available at: https://www.legislation.gov.uk/ukpga/2005/9/contents/enacted (Accessed 4 April 2023)

Nursing & Midwifery Council (2018). The code: professional standards of practice and behaviour for nurses, midwives and nursing associates. Available at: https://www.nmc.org.uk/globalassets/sitedocuments/nmc-publications/nmc-code.pdf (Accessed 28 February 2024).

18

Transforming Care and mental health support for people with a learning disability

Farzana Follows

This chapter introduces the Transforming Care programme within England, now known as the Learning Disability and Autism programme, with a focus on people at risk of admission to or in a mental health hospital. The programme has been providing guidance for organisations over the last decade and will continue to develop and advocate for positive change.

Transforming Care programme

The Transforming Care programme came about following the horrific abuse towards adults with a learning disability exposed by the BBC's *Panorama* programme at Winterbourne View hospital in May 2011. The events at Winterbourne View hospital triggered an in-depth review of care across England, including a programme of Care Quality Commission (CQC) inspections of 150 learning disability services as well as engagement by the Department of Health (DoH) to understand the experiences of people with a learning disability and autistic people, their families and carers, and organisations, professionals and providers that support them. The initial findings from this process were published in 2012 in an interim report by the DoH. The main findings are summarised below:

- Too many people were placed in mental health hospitals for assessment and treatment and were there longer than necessary.

- They were experiencing a model of care that went against published government guidance that people should have access to support and services they need locally, close to their family and friends.

- There was evidence of widespread poor quality of care, poor care planning, lack of meaningful activities in the day, and too much reliance on restraining people.

DOI: 10.4324/9781003341765-20

■ All parts of the system had a role in driving up standards, including commissioners of care, those who provide care and individual staff, the regulators and government.

Transforming Care: A National Response to Winterbourne View was then published (DoH, 2012a) and began a programme of work referred to as the Transforming Care programme. The aim of the programme is to ensure people with learning disability and autistic people who may also have challenging behaviour, including those with a mental health condition, receive appropriate specialist local community-based care, therefore shifting from a reliance on inpatient care.

Building the Right Support (Local Government Association, Association of Directors of Adult Social Services and NHS England, 2015) was published as part of the programme and introduced a national 'Service Model' informing what good services for people with a learning disability and autistic people should look like based on nine key principles (see Figure 18.1).

Further guidance was provided to commissioners to support the implementation of the national 'Service Model' by providing model service specifications for enhanced intensive support, community-based forensic support and for acute learning disability inpatient services (NHS England, 2017). The core functions of these services are presented below:

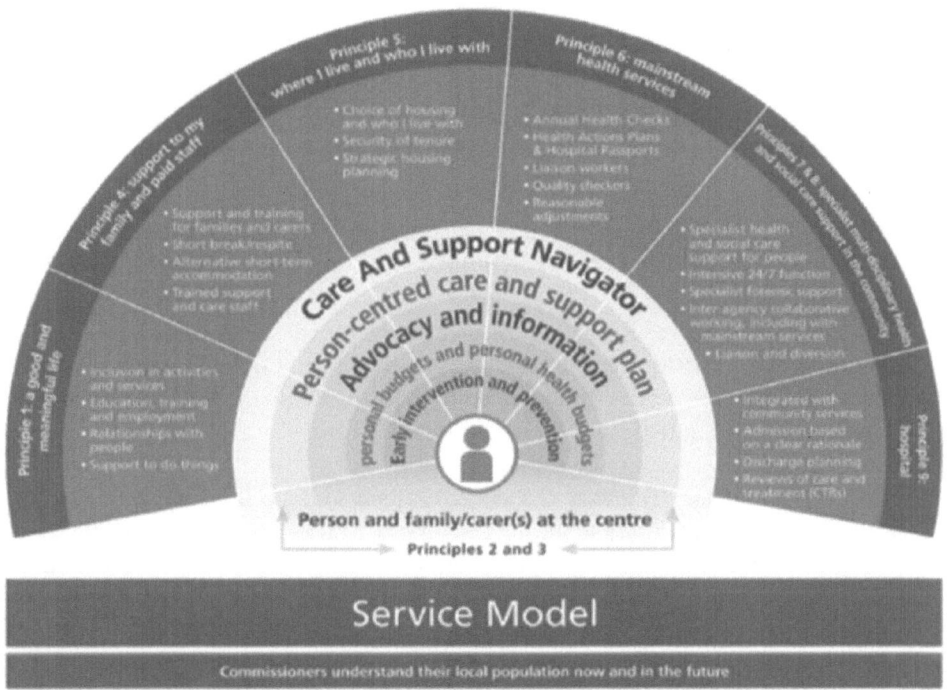

FIGURE 18.1 National Service Model for Transforming Care (NHS England, 2017)

Enhanced intensive support (four core functions):

- Assessment, treatment and support for individuals who display behaviour that challenges
- Provision of support and person specific training for other agencies supporting those individuals
- Coordination of transition from inpatient and other settings
- Crisis response.

Community-based forensic support (six core functions):

- Forensic risk assessment and management of risk in the community to ensure public safety and safety of the individual
- Delivery of offence-specific therapeutic interventions (e.g. to prevent sexual/violent offences)
- Case management of the most complex cases
- Support and training to other agencies providing day-to-day support to this group
- Consultancy and advice to system partners
- In-reach support to ensure safe and timely discharge.

Acute learning disability inpatient services (three core functions):

- Assessment (including for potential mental illness) of the causes of challenging behaviour, where it cannot be safely carried out in the community
- Treatment of mental illness where this is the cause of challenging behaviour (complemented by other interventions as appropriate), where it cannot be safely carried out in the community
- Reintegration of the individual back into the community after hospital treatment including provision of support/guidance to families and support providers.

Transforming Care Partnerships were developed across England made up of Clinical Commissioning Groups, local authorities and NHS England's specialised commissioners, to work in partnership with individuals with a learning disability and/or who are autistic and their families and carers in delivering local plans for the programme.

The NHS Long Term Plan (NHS, 2019) pledged a commitment to do more across the NHS to support people with a learning disability and autistic people to live happier, healthier and longer lives, and reinforce the work set out by the Transforming Care programme. The pledge includes:

- An increase in investment in intensive, crisis and forensic community care to ensure people receive tailored support in the community, as close to home as possible, and therefore reducing unnecessary admissions to mental health hospitals.

- A reduction in the number of people in inpatient services; therefore for every million adults there will be no more than 30 people with a learning disability and/or autism cared for in inpatient services and for children and young people with a learning disability and/or autism no more than 12 to 15 children per million.

- A keyworker for all children and young people with a learning disability and autistic people with the most complex needs by 2023/24, implementing the recommendation made by Dame Christine Lenehan in *These Are Our Children* (DoH, 2017), https://assets.publishing.service.gov.uk/government/uploads/system/uploads/attachment_data/file/585376/Lenehan_Review_Report.pdf

- To focus on improving the quality of inpatient care across the NHS as well as the independent sector by:

  - Ensuring all care commissioned by the NHS will need to have met the 'Learning Disability Improvement Standards' by 2023/24 (NHS Improvement, 2018).

  - Working with the CQC to implement recommendations on reducing the use of seclusion, long-term segregation and restraint for all patients in mental health hospitals, for children and young people in particular (see Joint Committee on Human Rights report on the Detention of Young People with Learning Disabilities and/or Autism (2019) and the government response (2020)).

  - Reducing the length of time people stay in mental health hospitals and support earlier transfers from inpatient settings. All areas will be monitored against a '12-point discharge plan' to support timely and effective discharges.

  - Reviewing and strengthening Care (Education) and Treatment Reviews, working in collaboration with people with a learning disability and autistic people, families and clinicians to evaluate their effectiveness in supporting unnecessary admissions and supporting discharge planning.

Care (Education) and Treatment Reviews (C(E)TRs)

C(E)TRs are relevant to people of all ages with a learning disability and autistic people who are either at risk of an admission to or are a patient in a mental health hospital. CTRs are for adult adults and C(E)TRs are for children and young people. They were introduced by NHS England as part of the Transforming Care programme to bring additional scrutiny and challenge to existing review processes, by identifying barriers to progress and making clear and constructive recommendations of how these may be overcome, therefore supporting the overall cause of reducing unnecessary admissions and lengthy stays in mental health hospitals. C(E)TRs are being driven by the NHS but the process involves local authorities and, where relevant, education services to ensure a more holistic approach, with the person and, where relevant, their family at the centre of care. C(E)TRs involve a panel: a chair (usually the responsible commissioner), an expert by experience (a person with a learning disability, or autistic person or a family carer with lived experience) and a clinical expert (a professional qualified to work in healthcare). The C(E)TR process is initiated when a person is identified as potentially at risk of admission to a mental health hospital. The C(E)TR supports a process of establishing whether the person requires an admission and whether their care and treatment can be met safely in the community with additional or alternative support and interventions. Where there are no alternatives, the process follows them through any subsequent admission, period of assessment and treatment and towards discharge. The first CTR policy was introduced in 2015 with the most recent revision of the policy being published in 2023: https://www.england.nhs.uk/wp-content/uploads/2023/01/Dynamic-support-register-and-Care-Education-and-Treatment-Review-policy-and-guide.pdf. NHS England also provides guidance and tools, including templates that contain Key Lines of Enquiry to guide and structure C(E)TRs for commissioners, panel members and people providing care: https://www.england.nhs.uk/learning-disabilities/care/ctr/commissioners/.

The latest policy combines with the requirement for Dynamic Support Registers to reflect an approach that does not see either of these as existing in isolation.

Dynamic Support Registers

Building the Right Support (2015) and the C(E)TR policy and guidance (2017) asked that local health commissioners work with their local partners, including social care and education, to develop and maintain a register of people (all age) with a learning disability and autistic people with increasing and/or complex care needs who may require additional support in the community as a safe and viable alternative to a mental health hospital. The register is now known as the dynamic support register (DSR).

DSRs are the mechanism for local systems to:

- use risk stratification to identify people at risk of admission to a mental health hospital
- work together to review the needs of each person registered on the DSR
- mobilise the right support (e.g. offer of a community C(E)TR, offer of a key-worker for children and young people, extra support at home) to help prevent the person being admitted to a mental health hospital.

DSRs also support with reviewing commissioning plans, financial plans and service delivery and development.

Local Area Emergency Protocol (LAEP)

The DSR and C(E)TR policy and guidance (NHS England, 2023) informs that ideally services should be fully aware of potential admissions well in advance via pre-planned community C(E)TRs and from information on their DSRs.

Where this has not occurred and an urgent admission is being contemplated, and where there is no time to organise a community C(E)TR, then a LAEP meeting is held (often by teleconference/video conference). This is where key individuals, e.g. members of the clinical team, senior health and social care service managers, advocate and care provider, meet to hold an urgent discussion. Every effort is also made to include the person and family/carers where possible. The purpose of the discussion is to provide additional scrutiny and challenge, reviewing the reason for hospital admission being sought and discussing any viable alternative options. A LAEP does not replace a community C(E)TR and should only be used by exception. If DSRs are effective, LAEPs will be rare and exceptional.

Consent

A C(E)TR cannot go ahead without the person's informed consent. This also applies to placing someone on a DSR. Consent needs to be formally documented. NHS England provide documents, 'My CTR Booklet' and 'My CTR Planner', that can be used to support informed consent: https://www.england.nhs.uk/learning-disabilities/care/ctr/commissioners/. If a person lacks mental capacity, informed consent must be gained from someone with parental responsibility where relevant, or holder of a valid and relevant Lasting Power of Attorney or a court appointed health and welfare deputy. If there is no lawful representative, a best interests decision needs to be made, applying the Mental Capacity Act (2005) and its Code of Practice. For people who have fluctuating mental capacity, their capacity 'at the material time' of the decision should be assessed. Any assessment of mental capacity is decision and purpose specific, in this case it only relates to the DSR or C(E)TR. People who lack mental capacity should still be as fully involved as possible in decisions about their care.

Assurance and oversight panels

NHS England recognise that despite holding C(E)TRs, for some people their length of stay can be long and/or restrictive and sometimes discharge is delayed. Therefore, there is now an expectation that each Integrated Care System (ICS) maintains an oversight panel to review care further that includes a learning disability and autism senior responsible officer/named executive lead, at least one expert by experience a medical director, a social care/local authority senior representative, commissioning representation and a senior clinician with expertise in learning disability and autism. The panel needs to also take into account quality assurance intelligence such as host commissioner reports and safeguarding information. The panel must take ownership of any actions from the review, escalate any issues that cannot be addressed at the ICS level to the relevant regional teams and provide evidence of how findings from reviews feed into the ICS delivery plan. Panels need to convene quarterly as a minimum and should review the C(E)TRs of people for whom concern has been expressed. This group includes, but not exclusive to, the following people:

- for children and young people with a stay of six months or longer
- for adults with a stay 12 months or longer (unless restricted by the Ministry of Justice)
- in long-term segregation or who are regularly secluded or subject to very restrictive practices
- who are placed in units or wards that CQC rates as inadequate
- who have made complaints about care, or their family has, and these have not been resolved to the satisfaction of all involved
- for whom a safeguarding referral has been made
- who have requested escalation or their family has
- where the responsible clinician has requested escalation
- where the responsible commissioner has requested escalation
- where the advocate has requested escalation
- who have declined a C(E)TR on two or more occasions.

Draft Mental Health Bill

In June 2022, the government published the Draft Mental Health Bill. The draft Bill would amend the criteria for detention under the Act so learning disability and autism would not be conditions for which a person could be subject to longer-term detention for treatment (section 3). This would mean people with a learning disability or autistic people could only be detained for treatment if they are suffering from a co-occurring mental disorder. The changes would not apply however to patients in the criminal justice system.

Measures in the draft Bill would also place C(E)TRs on a statutory footing.

'Building the Right Support Action Plan' was also published in 2022 with further focus on developing community services and reducing the reliance on inpatient care. https://www.gov.uk/government/publications/building-the-right-support-for-people-with-a-learning-disability-and-autistic-people/building-the-right-support-action-plan

Unfortunately, since Winterbourne View, the criminal abuse towards people with a learning disability remains a concern and there is still much to be done to get services right both in the community and in mental health hospitals. See Chapter 20 by Andrew McDonnell titled 'Undercover Documentaries: an Insider View' for more information relating to these and the care and treatment being provided:

- Whorlton Hall Hospital (2019): Undercover BBC filming showed hospital staff intimidating, mocking and restraining patients.

- Cygnet Yew Trees Hospital (2020): CCTV footage of patients being physically and emotionally abused.

- Eldertree Lodge (2021): CCTV footage of staff demonstrating ill-treatment or abuse and the use of inappropriate restrictive techniques.

- Cawston Park Hospital (2021): Significant failures found in the care of three adults with a learning disability who died.

- Breightmet Hospital (2023): The CQC found vulnerable adults being cared for at the hospital were not protected from abuse and poor care.

Think point

How does the programme support the prevention of abuse towards people with a learning disability in a mental health hospital? What would you do if you witnessed ill-treatment of patients? How do current and emerging policies such as the Transforming Care programme support your practice?

Reflection from the author and editors

The Transforming Care programme (Learning Disability and Autism programme) is about improving health and care services so that people can live meaningfully in the community with the right support and close to home. It is about preventing unnecessary admissions to mental health hospitals and, if admission is required, ensuring people receive good-quality care and do not remain in hospital longer than necessary. Although the programme has come a long way there is still much to be achieved in getting services right both in the community and in mental health hospitals which means that policy will inevitably change and move forward. Transforming Care will have its long-lasting seminal place within the timeline of policy and change for people with a learning disability and those who care for and support them (just as those before it including Community Care Act 1990, Valuing People 2001, Strengthening the Commitment 2012, have influenced the author's and editors' practice today). As learning disability nurses we have a key role to play in supporting the aims of the programme by ensuring the needs of people with a learning disability are understood by services, their human rights protected and barriers to receiving care are challenged and overcome.

References

Council for Disabled Children (2017) *These Are Our Children. A Review by Dame Christine Lenehan Director, Council for Disabled Children.* https://assets.publishing.service.gov.uk/government/uploads/system/uploads/attachment_data/file/585376/Lenehan_Review_Report.pdf

CTR guidance and tools for commissioners, panels and people providing care: https://www.england.nhs.uk/learning-disabilities/care/ctr/commissioners/

Department of Health (2012a) *Transforming Care: A National Response to Winterbourne View Hospital. Department of Health Review: Final Report.* http://assets.publishing.service.gov.uk/government/uploads/system/uploads/attachment_data/file/213215/final-report.pdf

Department of Health (2012b) *Winterbourne View Hospital Interim Report: Improving Care of Vulnerable People with Learning Disabilities.* Available at: http://www.dh.gov.uk/health/2012/06/interimwinterbourne/

Department of Health and Social Care (2020) *The Government Response to the Joint Committee on Human Rights Reports on the Detention of Young People with Learning Disabilities and/or Autism and the Implications of the Government's COVID-19 Response* https://www.gov.uk/government/publications/jchr-reports-on-the-detention-of-young-people-with-learning-disabilities-or-autism-government-response/the-government-response-to-the-joint-committee-on-human-rights-reports-on-the-detention-of-young-people-with-learning-disabilities-andor-autism-and-t

Department of Health and Social Care (2022) *Building the Right Support Action Plan* https://www.gov.uk/government/publications/building-the-right-support-for-people-with-a-learning-disability-and-autistic-people/building-the-right-support-action-plan

Draft Mental Health Bill (2022) https://www.gov.uk/government/publications/draft-mental-health-bill-2022

Joint Committee on Human Rights (2019) *The Detention of Young People with Learning Disabilities and/or Autism.* https://publications.parliament.uk/pa/jt201919/jtselect/jtrights/121/121.pdf

Local Government Association, Directors of Adult Social Services and NHS England (2015) Building the Right Support. A National Plan to Develop Community Services and Close Inpatient Facilities for People with a Learning Disability and/or Autism who Display Behaviour that Challenges, Including Those with a Mental Health Condition. https://www.england.nhs.uk/wp-content/uploads/2015/10/ld-nat-imp-plan-oct15.pdf

NHS (2019) *The NHS Long Term Plan.* https://www.longtermplan.nhs.uk/wp-content/uploads/2019/08/nhs-long-term-plan-version-1.2.pdf

NHS England (2017) *Care and Treatment Reviews (CTRs): Policy and Guidance Including Policy and Guidance on Care, Education and Treatment Reviews (CETRs) for Children and Young People.* https://www.proceduresonline.com/trixcms1/media/1524/care-and-treatment-reviews-policy-and-guidance.pdf

NHS England (2017) *Transforming Care. Model Service Specifications: Supporting Implementation of the Service Model.* https://www.england.nhs.uk/wp-content/uploads/2017/02/model-service-spec-2017.pdf

NHS England (2023) *Dynamic Support Register and Care (Education) and Treatment Review Policy and Guidance* https://www.england.nhs.uk/publication/dynamic-support-register-and-care-education-and-treatment-review-policy-and-guide/#heading-1

NHS Improvement (2018) *The Learning Disability Improvement Standards for NHS Trusts* https://www.england.nhs.uk/wp-content/uploads/2020/08/v1.17_Improvement_Standards_added_note.pdf

Case Examples

Whorlton Hall Hospital: https://www.bbc.co.uk/news/health-48367071

Cygnet Yew Trees Hospital: https://www.independent.co.uk/news/uk/crime/police-hospital-abuse-scandal-essex-cygnet-yew-trees-b572284.html

Eldertree Lodge: https://www.bbc.co.uk/news/uk-england-stoke-staffordshire-57503043

Cawston Park Hospital: https://www.bbc.co.uk/news/uk-england-norfolk-58466839

Breightmet Hospital: https://www.manchestereveningnews.co.uk/news/greater-manchester-news/inspectors-find-patients-severe-autism-24778941

19

An exploration of the Equality Act and making reasonable adjustments

Andrea Page, Helen Jones, Sally-Anne Dicken and Samantha Salmon

This section is supported by a case study and a PowerPoint presentation which we have included in the resources section of the book's webpage, free for all to download. Available from www.routledge.com/9781032377582

What is the Equality Act and what are reasonable adjustments?

Equality is ensuring that every individual has an equal opportunity to make the most of their lives and talents. No one should have poorer life chances because of the way that they were born, where they came from, what they believe or whether they have a disability.

The Equality Act (2010) (Gov.uk, 2010) https://www.gov.uk/guidance/equality-act-2010-guidance is a *comprehensive law* that aims to deal with all aspects of discrimination on the grounds of age, disability, gender, sexual orientation, marital status, ethnic background, religion and belief. This Act is 'anticipatory' meaning that services, organisations and nurses need to be proactive and think in advance about the types of adjustments people with a learning disability may need rather than wait until a problem arises.

Comprehensive law means that the Equality Act (2010) is detailed, broad in scope and content. It is a single legal framework with clear law to better tackle disadvantage and discrimination in the United Kingdom, including healthcare services. This act sets out a duty for public services to make reasonable adjustments, as far as possible so that disabled people are not disadvantaged in using these services; in other words a law to make sure people are treated fairly. What is defined as reasonable depends on several factors, such as if the change requested would address the disadvantage that disabled people experience, the practicability of making the

DOI: 10.4324/9781003341765-21

changes, the size of the service or organisation, the cost of making changes and the resources available for this and whether any changes have already been made.

How do they work?

The Equality Act (2010) describes three main methods for providing reasonable adjustments:

- Changing a practice, policy or procedure that has been identified as challenging for disabled people to access or use that service(s); for example, using simpler language and avoiding abbreviations and jargon, allowing extra time for appointments, inviting people to pre-admission visits so that they can familiarise themselves with the environment and know what to expect, giving people appointments at the start or end of clinics when the environment is less busy, changing the length of the appointment so that they have time to understand and communicate, ensure patients are first on the theatre list to reduce their waiting time, arranging for multiple procedures to be carried out under one general anaesthetic, ensuring that someone who knows the individual well is present at appointments, asking whether the person with a learning disability has a hospital passport and reading this key information, using short and clear instructions

- Changing a physical feature to remove, change, or to provide a reasonable method of avoiding barriers; for example, installing ramps, wider doors, accessible signage, changing places toilets, providing a quiet waiting area, changing the room temperature, removing distractions from a room, adjusting lighting in a room

- Providing additional aids or services where it would assist disabled people; for example, using British Sign Language interpreters, or providing information in an alternative format (Makaton, using symbols such as Widget or Talking Mats, social stories), providing a menu in an easy-read format to enable food choices in the same way as other patients be made.

Are there any differences in application across the UK?

Yes, whilst the Equality Act (2010) is a comprehensive law in England, Wales and Scotland. In Northern Ireland, disability discrimination is covered by the Disability Discrimination Act (1995) and the Northern Ireland Act (1998), which places a statutory obligation on public authorities to carry out their activities with due regard to the need to promote equality.

What is the importance for people with a learning disability and how are 'we' doing with this?

According to Learning Disabilities Mortality Review, which in 2021 was renamed as Learning from Life and Death Reviews (LeDeR): Action from Learning Report 2022/21 (NHS England 2021), on average, people with a learning disability and those with autism die earlier than the general population, and do not receive the same quality of care as people without a learning disability or who do not have autism. This resonates with the findings of the Care Quality Commission in (2022). Heslop at al. (2019) stated that of the deaths reviewed by the Learning Disability Mortality Review programme (LeDeR), 7% may have resulted from a lack of access to cancer screening and other gaps on service provision. Tuffrey-Wijne et al. (2014) in their mixed-methods study identified that there was a lack of effective systems for identifying and flagging that the person has a learning disability and their need for reasonable adjustments was therefore a significant barrier to the provision of reasonable adjustments in hospital. People with learning disabilities are more likely than the general population to experience multiple comorbidities and chronic health problems (Public Health England, 2018; Philips, 2019). Kinnear et al. (2018) in their cross-sectional study found that 98.7% of people with learning disabilities have two or more diagnoses in addition to having a learning disability which meant that they were more likely to access healthcare services and be admitted to hospital.

It is important that reiterate here that reasonable adjustments are personal. Pearce (2022: 15) includes comments from the RCN professional lead for learning disabilities Jonathon Beebee in her article, who makes the following important comment:

> You can't say: 'we've produced an easy read leaflet and that means our service is now accessible to people with learning disabilities'…instead, you need to think about what the person needs when they are entering a service to ensure they have equality of access. The starting point is always to ask the person or whoever is supporting them 'what they need and how can the service help'.

This perspective is stressed by Heslop et al. (2019) who state that it is essential to anticipate and support holistic needs of disabled people to access healthcare services and reduce the health inequalities that they experience. To do this Heslop et al. (2019) advocate that we learn from examples that have worked well, because these examples can be inspirational and allow others to gain an understanding of how solutions were considered, planned and implemented.

Marsden and Giles (2017), Heslop et al. (2019), Philips (2019), Ainsworth, Ainsworth and Blair (2021), George, Salloway and Welsh (2022) all agree that the communication needs of people with a learning disability are important when considering access to healthcare services, especially as evidence suggests that 50–90% of people with a learning disability in the UK have communication difficulties (RCSLT, 2019). This means that they may have additional support needs and may have difficulties understanding and remembering information. There are various tools and services available to help communication adjustments to be made, these include using interpreting services and paying particular attention to how the person expresses pain (Marsden and Giles, 2017). Hospital passports are meant to be standardised documents which contain information required to support the person in hospital, such as information about their illness, health, their likes, dislikes, the way the person communicates, how they indicate choices, the amount of physical contact they are okay with, interests, what reasonable adjustments they might need (Heslop et al., 2019; Philips, 2019). Northway et al. (2017) identified that there was considerable variation in the hospital passports in use within the UK which may limit their effectiveness; for example potential key information being missing; too much information being provided or vital information is not easy to find within the document. There is a need for a greater standardisation of hospital passports to address the issues this research identified.

A case study and teaching resource example

Lizzie – scenario

Lizzie is 35 and has profound and multiple learning disability. She is in hospital for a minor procedure under general anaesthetic later today. The doctor has requested observations particularly pulse, respiration and blood pressure before he will agree to this procedure being actioned.

Lizzie came in with her elderly mother a few hours ago, and they have both been left in the waiting area until now. Her mother has gone off for a much-needed break, and to get a drink.

Consider how you would spend time with Lizzie to ascertain her pulse, respiration and blood pressure.

Things to consider – and for discussion:

Carer stress, and involvement in the care and supervision when in hospital.

Lizzie's understanding, how to communicate with her. Use of communication aids, easy-read information.

Capacity and consent.

Involvement of wider multidisciplinary team, in particular learning disability nurses in preparation – prior to planned hospital admission.

Notes: Lizzie does exhibit self-injurious behaviour when she is unhappy. In the teaching session we would use an actor or role-player to respond to tone and approach and not allow touch unless feeling very comfortable with student. Maybe non-verbal or echolalic, using only one or two words.

Equipment required: Bubble tube and fibre-optics. Blood pressure machine, recording charts, communication passports, books without words, easy-read material. Please refer to the PowerPoint which can be downloaded from the resource section of this book's webpage (www.routledge.com/9781032377582). This PowerPoint gives tips on how to complete this case study and an insight into how this case study works as a teaching resource.

Example from practice

The Sensory Pod has been developed and brought to market by Murrays Medical Equipment Ltd, based in Dublin, Ireland and with a UK branch in Bromsgrove, Worcestershire. The Sensory Pod was conceived by Robert Byrne, an employee of Murrays, in 2017. The original idea was to provide a calming space for one of his children with autism as he found the alternatives very costly and requiring a lot of space, which was not available at home. Murray's arranged a trial in a special needs schools for a number of months. The initial feedback was extremely positive with occupational therapists and carers noting the immediate benefits when calming aroused children. The school started to incorporate it into the daily routine of some of the children, for example spending a short period of time in the Sensory Pod first thing each morning. They recorded an immediate reduction in striking incidents with staff after the child had relaxed in the Sensory Pod.

At the beginning of the chapter, we explored what the term 'reasonable adjustments' means, but why is this so important to patient care? This is Sally-Ann's perspective:

People with a learning disability experience poorer health and die significantly earlier than the general population; these differences in health status are recognised as a health inequality. There are numerous factors that may improve the health outcomes of people with learning disability.

Health inequalities can be the result of several different factors that exist across a range of dimensions, such as socio-economic deprivation and personal characteristics like age and sex. For example, in England, people living in the least deprived areas of the country live around 20 years longer in good health than people in the most deprived areas (Connolly, Baker and Fellows, 2017).

The LeDeR Review (Learning from Life and Death Reviews) (2021) found 6 out of 10 people with a learning disability died before they were 65. This compares to around 1 in 10 of the general population. There was also a regional difference between avoidable death for people with a learning disability, with the highest rate of 54% in the northwest compared to 42% in the southwest.

The causes of avoidable deaths for people with a learning disability reported in the LeDeR Review (2021) showed that 8% were linked to cancer, 14% due to hypertension, 17% due to diabetes and 17% to respiratory conditions.

Under the Equality Act (2010) health facilities have a duty to tackle inequalities by implementing reasonable adjustments so that people with a disability are not at a disadvantage.

The Care Quality Commission, 'Experiences of being in hospital for people with a learning disability and autistic people' (2022), found that people with a learning disability had positive and negative experiences when it came to having reasonable adjustments within hospital; the overall outcome was that the quality of care and treatment still needs improvement due to lack of skill, knowledge, time, continuity of care, patients and families being involved in their care and decisions

Placement experience of implementing a reasonable adjustment

From my own personal experiences when I was a learning disability student nurse on placement, I was asked to put together a blood desensitisation pack.

So, what is desensitisation? McLeod (2024) defines desensitisation as the reduction of fear or anxiety through the gradual exposure to the cause over a period of time. Desensitisation is a reasonable adjustment to support people to achieve having blood work completed without the use of restrictive interventions and enhance their understanding of why the blood test was requested.

The desensitisation pack that I put together includes environmental, sensory and communication, strategies to reduce anxiety and a step-by-step guide of a process to introduce having blood taken. The process is completed on the time scale of the patient. For example, a patient didn't like to do any activities in the morning and preferred interaction in the afternoon.

When the pack was completed and used in a community setting by myself and colleagues it was evident that the guide was too in-depth and that healthcare professionals, family members and the community team found the guide too big.

With this feedback and also using the tool myself I put together an assessment tool and pathway so that it not only met the needs of the patient but also the person that was supporting them. It's important to recognise that we have to consider reasonable adjustments for everyone involved in the care of the patient so we can achieve the best possible outcome.

We also have to accept that desensitisation may not work initially for some people, in these cases we still have a duty to look for other options when possible before deciding on either a restrictive method or not doing anything at this time.

Another example within my practice is of a patient who could not tolerate desensitisation or any procedure for his health. This meant that chemical restriction was considered, using 'best interest' decision-making processes and a capacity assessment. We were aware that there had been no blood test taken to check cholesterol and glucose levels which was required given the medications they were taking. After discussing with everyone involved and due to the low dose of medication prescribed, it was agreed to be in this individual's best interest not to have a blood test due to the impact it would have on the patient and also the impact of chemical restraint. As part of our reasonable adjustments we ensured that this patient would still be monitored for any side effects from the medication and we agreed that his blood pressure and weight would be monitored. At this stage, we began the process of desensitisation around blood pressure with him.

As a student and now a practising nurse we have moral duty to our patients, their family and ourselves to always explore every possible avenue so that they can live a long and healthy life and that is why the Equality Act and reasonable adjustments are so crucial.

Useful organisations

https://www.easyhealth.org.uk/ An online library of accessible health information with over 390 resources in video and leaflet formats, covering 120 health conditions or topics, including abdominal cancer, annual health checks, back pain, blood tests, breast checks, hospital passports, nurses, smear tests, surgery, ultrasound scans and X-rays. Membership is free (date accessed 13.10.2022).

https://makaton.org Makaton is a language programme that uses symbols, signs and speech to enable people to communicate (date accessed 12.10.2022).

https://www.mencap.org.uk/advice-and-support/health-coronavirus/health-guides Provides support for the person with a learning disability if going into hospital – overview of hospital passports, the learning disability register, reasonable adjustments (date accessed 18.10.2022).

https://murraysmedical.co.uk Each Sensory Pod measures 8 foot wide x 4 foot deep x 6 foot high, comes with speakers for calming music, LED lighting in five colours for the interior to allow the user to select the most relaxing colour for their needs. The door slides over to cocoon the child, or it can be left open if desired. When the door is closed there is a viewing screen to provide child protection for both child and adult. It comes in a white, easy clean ABS plastic shell, which looks futuristic or there is an option of a themed wrap, like to make the Sensory Pod more welcoming to children. The reasoning behind these improvements was to mimic the feel of complete sensory rooms within the space of a Sensory Pod.

https://www.nhs.uk/conditions/learning-disabilities/going-into-hospital/ Provides support for the person with a learning disability if going into hospital – overview of hospital passports (date accessed 18.10.2022).

https://www.stoswoldsuk.org Distress and Discomfort Assessment Tool also known as the Disability Distress Assessment Tool (DisDAT). This aims to identify distress cues in people with severely limited communication (date accessed 12.10.2022).

https://www.talkingmats.com Talking Mats is an interactive resource that uses symbols to help people with communication difficulties by increasing their capacity to think about and express views about things that matter to them. This resource has a strong evidence base and is particularly useful when obtaining consent for treatments (date accessed 12.10.2022).

https://widget.com Symbols to help people read, understand and communicate. This is a software package to create visual support for documents (date accessed 12.10.2022).

References

Ainsworth, V., Ainsworth, T. and Blair, J. (2021) How to get it right for people with learning disabilities in the emergency department: ask and engage. *Emergency Nurse*, 29(2), 32–41. doi: 10.7748/en.2021.e2070

Barber, C. (2022) *Learning Disabilities: A Non-Specialist Introduction for Nursing, Health and Social Care*. Banbury: Lantern Publishing.

Beresford, C.J. (2022) Supporting people with learning disabilities to manage their diabetes with insulin. *Journal of Diabetes Nursing* 26(3), 1–5.

Care Quality Commission (CQC) (2022) Experiences of being in hospital for people with a learning disability and autistic people. https://www.cqc.org.uk/publication/experiences-being-hospital-people-learning-disability-and-autistic-people (date accessed 8.11.2022)

Connolly, A., Baker, A. and Fellows, C. (2017) Understanding health inequalities in England https://ukhsa.blog.gov.uk/2017/07/13/understanding-health-inequalities-in-england/ (date accessed 2.2.2023)

George, S., Salloway, R. & Welsh, K. (2022) Making reasonable adjustments to cancer services for people with learning disabilities. *Cancer Nursing Practice*, 21(5), 35–41.

Heslop, P., Calkin, R., Huxor, A., Byrne, V. and Gielnik, K. (2018) The learning disabilities mortality review (LeDeR) programme annual report 2018. University of Bristol. https://www.bristol.ac.uk/media-library/sites/sps/leder/LeDeR_Annual_Report_2018%20published%20May%202019.pdf (date accessed 13.10.2022)

Heslop, P., Turner, S., Read, S., Tucker, J., Seaton, S. and Evans, B. (2019) Implementing reasonable adjustments for disabled people in healthcare services. *Nursing Standard*, 34(8), 29–34. https://doi.org/10.7748/ns.2019.e11172

Kinnear, D., Morrison, J., Allan, L., Henderson, A., Smiley, E. and Cooper, S.A. (2018) Prevalence of physical conditions and multimorbidity in a cohort of adults with intellectual disabilities with and without Down syndrome: cross-sectional study. *BMJ Open*, 5 February, 8(2): e018292. doi: 10.1136/bmjopen-2017-018292. PMID: 29431619; PMCID: PMC5829598.

Learning from Life and Death Reviews (LeDeR) (2021) https://www.england.nhs.uk/learning-disabilities/improving-health/learning-from-lives-and-deaths/ (date accessed 2.2.2023)

Marsden, D. and Giles, R. (2017) The 4C framework for making reasonable adjustments for people with learning disabilities. *Nursing Standard*, 31(21), 45–53.

McLeod, S. (2024) Systematic desensitization therapy in psychology. Retrieved from www.simplypsychology.org/systematic-Desensitisation.html (date accessed 9.1.2025)

NHS England (2021) Learning Disabilities Mortality Review (LeDeR): Action from Learning Report 2020/21 https://www.england.nhs.uk/publication/leder-action-from-learning-report-2021/ (date accessed 13.10.2022)

NHS.UK (2015) What is the Mental Capacity Act? – Care and support – NHS Choices. [online] Available at: Mental Capacity Act - NHS (www.nhs.uk) (date accessed 2.2.2023)

Northway, R., Rees, S., Davies, M. and Williams, S. (2017) Hospital passports, patient safety and person-centred care: A review of documents currently used for people with intellectual disabilities in the UK. *Journal of Clinical Nursing*. December, 26(23–24): 5160–5168. doi: 10.1111/jocn.14065.

Northway, R. and Hopes, P. (2022) *Learning Disability Nursing: Developing Professional Practice*. St Albans: Critical Publishing.

Pearce, L. (2022) Reasonable adjustments: What do I need to know? *Learning Disability Practice*, 25(3), 15–17.

Pearce, L. (2022) Reasonable adjustments: What do I need to know? *Learning Disability Practice*, 25(3), 15–17.

Philips, L. (2019) Learning disabilities: making reasonable adjustments in hospital. *Nursing Times*, 115(10), 38–42.

Public Health England (2018) Learning disabilities: applying All Our Health https://www.gov.uk/government/publications/learning-disability-applying-all-our-health/learning-disabilities-applying-all-our-health (date accessed 18.10.2022)

RCSLT (2019) Royal College of Speech and Language Therapists Conference 2019 https://www.rcslt.org/events/rcslt-conference-2019/

Trueland, J. (2022) How nurses can help reduce anxiety about healthcare appointments. *Learning Disability Practice*, 25(2), 11–13. doi: 10.7748/ldp.25.2.11.s4

Tuffrey-Wijne, I. Goulding, L., Giatras, N., Abraham, E., Gillard, S., White, S., Edwards, C., and Hollins, S. (2014) The barriers to and enablers of providing reasonably adjusted health services to people with intellectual disabilities in acute hospitals: evidence from a mixed-methods study. *BMJ Open*, April 16, 4(4): e004606. doi: 10.1136/bmjopen-2013-004606.

Whitehouse, C., Crossley, R., Copping, J., and Hall, H. (2021) Creating a Covid-19 vaccination clinic for people with learning disabilities. *Nursing Times* [online]; 117: 7, 23–26. https://cdn.ps.emap.com/wp-content/uploads/sites/3/2021/06/210623-Creating-a-Covid-19-vaccination-clinic-for-people-with-learning-disabilities.pdf (accessed 18.10.2022)

20

Undercover documentaries
An insider view

Andrew McDonnell

Abuse of people who are vulnerable, especially in institutional care, is not a new subject. In 1967, an inquiry was set up about Ely Hospital to investigate abuse of people in psychiatric care. There are so many examples that have occurred over the years that demonstrate a repeated pattern of staff members systematically abusing the vulnerable. Similar situations have occurred in services that support people with intellectual disabilities. In many of these cases, whistleblowers or undercover investigations have been required to bring these issues to the attention of the public. This chapter will focus on the role of undercover and exposé documentaries that often involve, directly and indirectly, nurses of different training and backgrounds. We will try to make sense of their usefulness and impact.

Historical context

Since the Ely Hospital inquiry, reported in 1969, there have been many others. In 1984, the author John Martin catalogued to that date a range of hospital-based investigations which focused primarily on abusive practices in care environments. The author, as a young assistant psychologist, spent a year in a hospital (Churchill House in Berkshire) that had two pages in John Martin's book. The first major undercover documentary that really focused on abusive practices was the investigation of Borocourt Hospital called *Silent Minority* (1981). Whilst it is only an opinion, the emotional impact of this early documentary was huge. In some ways, it could be argued that it was the death knell for hospitals for people with learning disabilities.

Undercover documentaries that focus on abusive practices have increased as a phenomenon over the last 20 years. The growth of social media has clearly been a factor, and public awareness can also be raised by high-profile reporting of negligent practice. Oliver McGowan was a young autistic man who died after being given anti-psychotic medication, despite medical staff being told repeatedly by both Oliver and his parents that he had reacted badly to it in the past. The drug caused his brain to swell severely and he died in intensive care. The Oliver McGowan

DOI: 10.4324/9781003341765-22

tragedy has led to actions that include the development of training in autism for what is described as tertiary or tier 4 services. The National Autism Training Programme (NATP) initiative by Georgia Pavlopoulou and colleagues is another step in the right direction.

Whilst it would be impossible to catalogue all of the inquiry documentaries that have occurred over the last two decades, we have had notable examples that cover both the private and public sector, some of which we will now look at in more detail.

A psychologist's view

As a clinical psychologist, I have had extensive experience and involvement with undercover documentaries in the UK. These documentaries are nearly all focused on abusive practices on vulnerable individuals with intellectual disabilities and/or autism. It is important to contextualise why we focus on tragedy as a learning mechanism. Undercover documentaries shed light on topics that people find taboo and uncomfortable.

The first documentary I was ever involved with was entitled *MacIntyre Undercover*, named after journalist Donal MacIntyre (BBC, 1999). This documentary focused on a private home for adults with learning disabilities in Kent. Abusive practices such as the excessive use of restraint were clearly identified by the journalists involved. This documentary did create additional controversy at the time as some journalists thought that the restraint issues had been over-sensationalised (Gibson, 2022). Compared to other documentaries, this one has had relatively little exposure in the more recent conversations about abusive practices. My experience of the BBC journalists was that they were highly professional, and they themselves seemed to be surprised that the abusive practices that they had uncovered appeared to have been 'normalised'.

The original MacIntyre documentary did affirm to me that, beyond the ideas of sensationalism, exposing bad practice and trying to get systemic change sometimes needs media-based interventions. A recent example of this at the time of writing is the documentaries and the drama *Mr Bates vs The Post Office* about the post office scandal, which clearly have had a huge impact on politicians today.

In 2011, I was approached by BBC *Panorama* to provide some expert front-of-screen commentary on abusive practices that involved excessive use of psychological punishment and restraint in an adult specialist service in the Bristol area called Winterbourne View. I was honoured to be asked to be one of two main experts (the other expert was the late Professor Jim Mansell, who was widely regarded as one of the leading authorities on disability care in the UK). Abusive practices had been exposed in a privately run care home called Winterbourne View which, at the time, was thought to be a specialist service for people with difficult behaviours and autism. The original release from the BBC described it as follows (2012):

> BBC One's *Panorama* showed patients at a residential care home near Bristol, being slapped and restrained under chairs, having their hair pulled and being held down as medication was forced into their mouths.

The victims, who had severe learning disabilities, were visibly upset and were shown screaming and shaking.

One victim was showered while fully clothed and had mouthwash poured into her eyes.

Undercover recordings showed one senior care worker at Winterbourne View asking a patient whether they wanted him to get a 'cheese grater and grate your face off?'

...

Dr Peter Carter, head of the Royal College of Nursing, said: 'The sickening abuse revealed in this programme is more shocking than anything we could have imagined.'

I remember when Professor Jim Mansell was asked about what should be done about Winterbourne View, he simply said, 'Close it.' Jim's views were also very clear that clustering people together who are distressed, as we often do in our healthcare models, made very little sense from a behavioural perspective.

This documentary for me personally was very difficult to process. The footage that I saw was distressing because at the time I did not know who these people were, or where the place was; I was simply asked to respond as an expert to specific video sequences. I remember having to take comfort breaks throughout the day. One of the film crew at the time remarked, 'Don't you guys get used to this stuff?' They simply got a one word reply, 'No.' My honest comment was, 'If I had got used to this stuff, I would be desensitised to it and no good at my job.'

The Winterbourne View documentary made a considerable impact, more than even I expected at the time. In 2013, MIND produced a report entitled *Mental Health Crisis Care: Physical Restraint in Crisis*. This report focused on the use of physical restraint in hospital settings in the UK (p. 8):

> Following the Winterbourne View investigation, the Care Quality Commission produced a briefing on restrictive practices in mental health and learning disability settings. It explored a programme of unannounced inspections of services, alongside evidence from visits to people detained under the Mental Health Act. Although the briefing identified the use of different types of restrictive practices, which are still prevalent, such as seclusion/segregation techniques, there was also evidence on the use of physical restraint varying in frequency and intensity with some inspection reports highlighting how common the practice was in some areas.

I do recall at the time that the documentary was aired that there was considerable consternation among my many colleagues that the BBC should have just given their evidence to the police, and not made the programme. I do not agree with such a perspective, although I understand it. My own experience of this documentary was that the journalists involved (some of whom are still in contact with the many families and individuals who were victims of these practices) understood that there was a responsibility to separate the aims of the documentary from any kind of investigatory process. In my own opinion, when I hear people say, 'Why don't they make documentaries about best practice in care?', the answer lies in the public and social media's thirst for negative information. More importantly, journalists have to have the right to hold people to account. The experience of being involved with such documentaries can be emotionally traumatising. To be totally frank and honest, whilst I believe that undercover documentaries will sadly have a role, after the Winterbourne View experience I made a personal vow that I would never appear on a documentary like that again. To the readers of this book, if there is one simple reflection, it is never make promises that you know you cannot keep.

In 2019, I was asked by BBC *Panorama* again to be involved in a similar undercover documentary with Professor Glynis Murphy, who was Professor Jim Mansell's successor at the Tizard Centre at the University of Kent. The documentary was entitled *Undercover Hospital Abuse Scandal* (*Panorama*, 2019), and looked at abusive practices by staff in Whorlton Hall. Journalist Olivia Davies went undercover, and revealed the mocking, taunting and intimidation of vulnerable adults. In January 2024, four members of staff involved in the documentary were prosecuted for mistreatment of vulnerable patients in their care (Jagger and Harris, 2024).

Why are people with learning disabilities often involved in these documentaries?

It would appear to be the case, based on predominantly anecdotal evidence, that people with learning disabilities as a population may attract more documentaries about abuse. Abuses of restraint and other restrictive practices do occur in other sectors, but why is it that vulnerable people with intellectual disabilities and autism are so often involved?

Emerging themes

Based on first-hand experience, there are clear themes to many of the undercover documentaries. Psychologically, members of the public witness practices of abuse that are very real and emotional for them. I would encourage the reader to look at the Winterbourne View BBC documentary, and the physical restraints used on Simone. Understanding the very real helplessness in those situations is a primary purpose of these documentaries. There are also clear psychological processes that are involved when examining the behaviour of staff in these documentaries.

Groupthink and social psychological explanations

Social psychological research has identified group-based factors that impact on human behaviour. The Milgram studies (1963) identified how far individuals would be prepared to go to give electric shocks to individuals in a contrived setting, mostly consisting of actors. In the classic Milgram experiment, members of the public were paid to participate in the study where they were told they were studying the effects of electric shocks on learning. They would then see an individual with an electrical device (the person being an actor), and would then be told the person had to learn some word sequences. If they made a mistake, the participant should administer a mild electric shock. In this series of studies, over a third of people administered what they believed to be quite severe shocks to individuals. These and many other studies do show that human beings who can be decent and law-abiding do seem to have a process of justifying even some of the most heinous acts. In the Winterbourne documentary, one of the participants said that they were going to be 'tough' on clients because it was 'for their own good'. Other psychologists have referred to the mechanism of what would be described as 'groupthink' (Tajfel, 1979). In this situation, people will justify their actions. In something called the Stanford Prison Experiment, students were participating as either prison guards or prisoners. It was explained to them that they would be in a mock prison situation, and that their behaviours were being monitored. The original study was meant to last two weeks, but it was abandoned after a few days due to distressed behaviours shown by the prisoners, and the early signs of abusive behaviours by the guards.

Similar studies have been repeated over the years which demonstrate clearly that we have almost an innate ability to justify our actions. When we apply this to the undercover documentaries, on repeated occasions examples of this 'groupthink' occur. It does raise an interesting question about whether these are people who are 'bad', or whether they are individuals who are just driven by circumstance. On a personal note, I genuinely believe that a small minority of individuals are attracted to working with the vulnerable for the wrong reasons. These are the types of individuals who almost gleefully exert control over other human beings. In the Winterbourne View documentary, the staff member 'Wayne' shows himself to be one of these individuals when at one point he was sitting on a chair placed on top of an individual called Simone.

Abuse of restrictive practices such as restraint and seclusion

The abuse of restraint and seclusion are also common themes. These types of methods of control are often described as 'a last resort' (Deveau and McDonnell, 2009). In practice, they can become overused by frontline staff almost as a form of punishment. When I use the term 'punishment', I refer to the definition used by Article 3 of the Council of Europe's European Convention on Human Rights given further effect in the Human Rights Act 1998, which states that no one shall be subjected to torture, inhuman or degrading treatment or punishment. It is easy after watching any undercover documentaries to think of the abusive practices in terms of victims and perpetrators. It is clear that such distinctions may inhibit people from developing an understanding of why abusive practices occur. I remember a personal comment from a leading expert after the Winterbourne View documentary, where that person quite clearly said, 'The staff in these situations are very stressed.' My response to that was to acknowledge that working with people in these situations is stressful, but that the vast majority of highly stressed staff, in my experience, do not commit acts of abuse.

The slippery slope to abuse

It is very clear to me that abusive practices, as witnessed in the Winterbourne View and Whorlton Hall documentaries, and many others, do not occur in a 'vacuum'. Dehumanisation and de-individuation (Zimbardo, 1969) are processes that occur over time. It is important to think about whether there are any early signs that could be recognise indicators that there is a potential for 'groupthink' and over-justification of punitive practices.

After the Winterbourne View documentary, I co-wrote a practitioner article for *Learning Disability Practice* called 'The Slippery Slope to Abuse' (McDonnell, Breen, Deveau, Goulding & Smyth, 2014). In this article, my colleagues and I identified that in the complex interactions between people with disabilities and staff who become 'abusers', there were a number of early signs. Although much of this is anecdotal in nature and based on experience, there are obvious indicators. The language that staff use about people – which can include making derogatory comments about individuals and inappropriate use of humour – would seem to be an indicator. Many of these comments can also lead to over-justification of what could best be described as minor restrictions and sanctions. In essence, people start to restrict access to things that give people pleasure, often making them conditional on good behaviour.

I have also experienced people overestimating purpose and deliberate intent to incidents of challenging behaviour. If you believe that someone is deliberately out to hurt you, it is highly likely that it will alter your behavioural responses to that person. It is now more commonly acknowledged that there are cognitive biases that have an impact on our responses to behaviour (Osgood, 2023). Developing empathy for an individual, but also understanding what has been referred to as the 'double empathy problem' (Milton, 2018), is important when considering how people respond to behaviours of concern.

Think point

Have a look at the 'double empathy problem' as described by Milton and consider what your interpretation of this is and possible implications for your practice.

The possibility of working with staff teams to become more aware of this bias at its early stages of development may be helpful. An example of this is when I have facilitated discussions about undercover documentaries with individuals to help them understand and develop empathy for individuals.

Changing policies and minds

Top-down approaches

Often when undercover documentaries expose bad practice, there are clearly ideas and suggestions for changing ideas and practices 'on-the-ground'. Just as important is to change policy and approaches. One key area is to provide regulation and guidance about what are often described as restrictive practices (restraint, seclusion, punitive sanctions). There has been a much greater emphasis on the reduction of restrictive practices in the UK in both health and social care environments. The emphasis on the 'least restrictive' responses has been a driving theme. Reducing restrictions requires both a top-down and bottom-up approach. Key issues sometimes need a statutory framework. The recent expert working party chaired by the same Baroness Hollins who was involved with the Winterbourne View expert analysis concluded that seclusion and long-term segregation should be referred to as 'solitary confinement', and that there was a requirement to change our mental health act legislation to assist in outlawing these practices (Department of Health and Social Care, 2023):

> Members are unanimous in recommending that all instances of enforced social isolation, including seclusion and long-term segregation, should be renamed 'solitary confinement'. The panel recommends that its use with children and young people under the age of 18 should be ended with immediate effect, and that the use of solitary confinement for people with a learning disability and/or autistic people should be severely curtailed and time limited. Minimum standards for the use of solitary confinement should be introduced urgently through amendments to the Mental Health Act 1983: Code of Practice.

At the time of writing, our current government appears to have not made space in parliamentary time to make the appropriate amendments to the Mental Health Code of Practice. This demonstrates that there is often a battle between frontline practitioners and policy makers. In my view, having a high threshold should lead to better standards. The recent example of Baroness Hollins shows that an evidence-based approach where politicians follow expert recommendations needs to be re-embraced if we are truly to reduce restrictive practices.

In the UK, the Restraint Reduction Network (RRN) has evolved into a body that is trying to develop further standards around the training of staff. It is very clear to me that guidance and regulations can always be strengthened. Implicit in guidance is that safety for all parties should be our primary goal. It is interesting to note that Abraham Maslow in his well-documented hierarchy of needs described safety as the fundamental foundation (Maslow, 1943).

Bottom-up approaches

Bottom-up approaches focus on equipping frontline staff with the necessary reflective skills to help prevent incidents of abuse. There are many obvious areas where training frontline staff and their leadership and coaching will be important. I admit a bias, and would suggest strongly that training staff in understanding neurodiverse conditions such as autism is a critical building block. In both Winterbourne View and Whorlton Hall, there is a consistent theme that abuse of people on the autistic spectrum by staff appears to show 'a lack of emotional connection'. Focusing on relationship building is critical in this process. The training of staff in de-escalation skills and appropriate physical intervention skills need to be placed in context of organisational cultures.

Bottom-up processes, similar to top-down processes, are both needed to effect change. It might be regarded as a slightly political point, but the perceived medical model of placing people together who are highly distressed appears to be a significant part of the problem. In many cases individuals are being detained as they represent a risk to themselves or others. Changing this model requires more of a top-down approach, as quite often undercover documentaries do tend to focus on these types of establishments.

Conclusion

This chapter outlines some of the key issues that are involved in improving our practice. We have examined examples such as Winterbourne View and individual cases of tragedy. Watch a number of these documentaries and reflect on what you would do in the future if you witnessed a situation like this. Reflective approaches are so important in this area; taking ownership and responsibility instead of justifying and minimising. Be conscious of the fact that many of the issues we have outlined are not just about abuse of power, but they involve fundamental human rights.

Note

There have been noticeable examples of restraint-related deaths in other sectors. Deaths in health and social care settings have been acknowledged to occur in the UK (Paterson, Bradley, Stark, Saddler, Leadbetter & Allen, 2003). Restraint-related deaths do not just occur in care settings, but in other contexts as well. The UK police and other agencies also report issues in this area.

One of the most harrowing deaths in psychiatric care in the UK involved the case of David 'Rocky' Bennett. In 2003, an independent inquiry report reported on the death of Bennett, who was a 38-year-old Afro-Caribbean patient with a diagnosis of schizophrenia who died in 1998. He died in a medium-secure unit in Norwich called the Norvic Clinic. He was held face-down on the floor by staff in response to his behaviour for almost 25 minutes by a team of five nurses. A later inquiry by Sir John Blofeld reported that he had sustained injuries under restraint due to the excessive force. In the investigation, it was revealed that the nurses did not release Mr Bennett from the hold until he 'went quiet'. Sir John Blofeld (a retired high court judge) identified institutional racism as a component in his death.

References

BBC. (1999). *MacIntyre Undercover: Care Homes*. BBC One.

BBC. (2012). Winterbourne View: Abuse footage shocked nation, BBC [Online]. Available from https://www.bbc.co.uk/news/uk-england-bristol-20084254.

Channel 4. (2023). Locked away: Our autism scandal *Dispatches*, Channel 4. Available from: https://www.channel4.com/programmes/locked-away-our-autism-scandal-dispatches/on-demand/73942-001.

Department of Health and Social Care. (2023). Baroness Hollins' final report: 'My heart breaks – s olitary confinement in hospital has no therapeutic benefit for people with a learning disability and autistic people', *Independent Care (Education) and Treatment Reviews: Final Report,*

2023. Available from https://www.gov.uk/government/publications/independent-care-education-and-treatment-reviews-final-report-2023/baroness-hollins-final-report-my-heart-breaks-solitary-confinement-in-hospital-has-no-therapeutic-benefit-for-people-with-a-learning-disability-an#additional-references-and-literature-review.

Deveau, R. & McDonnell, A. (2009). As the last resort: Reducing the use of restrictive physical interventions using organisational approaches. *British Journal of Learning Disabilities*, 37(3), 172–177.

Evans, N. (1981). *Silent Minority*, ITV. Available from https://www.youtube.com/watch?v=O4eqzf_e4u4.

Gibson, O. (2002). MacIntyre receives police apology. *The Guardian* [Online]. Available from https://www.theguardian.com/media/2002/oct/08/broadcasting.bbc4

Jagger, S. & Harris, P. (2024). Whorlton Hall: Four carers sentenced for abusing hospital patients, BBC [Online]. Available from https://www.bbc.co.uk/news/uk-england-tees-68021858.

Maslow, A. H. (1943). A theory of human motivation. *Psychological Review*, 50(4): 370–396. https://psycnet.apa.org/doi/10.1037/h0054346

McDonnell, A., Breen, E., Deveau, R., Goulding, E. & Smyth, J. (2014). How nurses and carers can avoid the slippery slope to abuse. *Learning Disability Practice*, 17(5): 36–39. doi: 10.7748/ldp.17.5.36.e1516.

Milgram, S. (1963). Behavioural study of obedience, *The Journal of Abnormal and Social Psychology*, 67(4): 371–378. doi:10.1037/h0040525.

MIND. (2013). Mental health crisis care: Physical restraint in crisis. A report on physical restraint in hospital settings in England, MIND. Available from: https://www.mind.org.uk/media-a/4378/physical_restraint_final_web_version.pdf.

Osgood, J.M. (2023). Targeting cognitive bias to reduce anger and aggression, in C.R. Martin, V.R. Preedy and V.B. Patel (eds) *Handbook of Anger, Aggression, and Violence*. Springer, Cham. https://doi.org/10.1007/978-3-031-31547-3_112

Panorama. (2011). Undercover care: The abuse exposed, *Panorama*, BBC One.

Panorama. (2019). Undercover hospital abuse scandal, *Panorama*, BBC One.

Paterson, B., Bradley, P., Stark, C., Saddler, D., Leadbetter, D., & Allen, D. (2003). Deaths associated with restraint use in health and social care in the UK. The results of a preliminary survey. *Journal of Psychiatric and Mental Health Nursing*, 10(1): 3–15. doi:10.1046/j.1365-2850.2003.00523.x.

Tajfel, H. (1979). Individuals and groups in social psychology. *British Journal of Social and Clinical Psychology*, 18(2), 183–190.

Zimbardo, P. G. (1969). The human choice: Individuation, reason, and order versus deindividuation, impulse, and chaos. *Nebraska Symposium on Motivation*, 17, 237–307.

Responding to inequality and inequity

We are nursing in an imperfect world

Nikita Garrick

During my nursing apprenticeship placement with a Health Facilitation acute liaison team in the West Midlands, I had the opportunity to visit several wards in a hospital to review the standards of care provided for patients with a learning disability. Upon my visit to the fourth ward, I requested to review a patient's nursing file to ascertain if the patient had a recent bowel movement and to establish if this information had been documented.

Within the nursing file, hospital staff had access to the patient's hospital passport, which is an international document designed to overcome communication barriers that may impede individuals with intellectual disabilities from receiving adequate medical care. Although the passport is believed to enhance patient safety and promote person-centred care, its implementation may differ in structure and effectiveness, potentially limiting its usefulness (Northway et al., 2017). The patient's medical record clearly indicated that they encountered regular constipation; their treatment includes maintaining a high-fibre diet and states they are taking regular prescription laxatives. On speaking to the ward nurse, I was informed they were unaware of what a hospital passport was. Furthermore, the department was uninformed that the patient had difficulty with bowel movements, as this information was not communicated during the patient's recent transfer from A&E. The ward nurse requested to see the hospital passport, as she was unaware it was situated within the patient's file. It was apparent the ward nurse was embarrassed while discussing the patient's constipation as this crucial need was almost overlooked. As documented, the patient had not experienced a bowel movement for several consecutive days. I requested that the patient be examined by a doctor to rule out the possibility of faecal impaction and to consider prescribing a course of laxatives. Untreated constipation can pose a serious risk to individuals with a learning disability, potentially leading to life-threatening consequences (NHS England, 2023a). Therefore, it is imperative to seek medical advice for the individual in your care to be assessed and prescribed the most appropriate treatment.

NHS England (2023d) LeDeR action from learning report states people with a learning disability are at greater risk of constipation. According to the report,

DOI: 10.4324/9781003341765-24

constipation was identified as among the top ten most reported chronic health conditions among individuals with a learning disability who died in 2020, accounting for 55% of cases. This suggests people with a learning disability die on average earlier than people without a learning disability, as they do not always receive the same quality of care. Which, given that constipation can be prevented and treated with medication, is extremely concerning (NHS, 2019). However, for people with learning disabilities to live longer, healthier and happier lives, it is necessary to implement what has been learned from LeDeR reviews to enhance treatment pathways and reduce inequalities in care, such as the 'Constipation campaign toolkit' available at: https://www.england.nhs.uk/long-read/constipation-campaign-toolkit/. The toolkit offers the following resources intended to be utilised within the home and care environment settings: QR code on a poster, social media posts, easy read leaflets and a short animation. These materials will explain the indicators of constipation with the aim of promoting timely intervention and improving outcomes for individuals with a learning disability who experience constipation (NHS England, 2023b).

Furthermore, while reviewing the patient's nursing file, I came across their Recommended Summary Plan for Emergency Care and Treatment (ReSPECT) document and observed that the reason for do not attempt cardiopulmonary resuscitation (DNACPR) was due to futility. Due to my unfamiliarity with the definition of this word, my practice assessor advised that I conduct research on it. The definition of the word 'pointless' or 'useless' astounded me, as I believed it implied that the patient's existence lacked purpose due to their learning disability. However, one way of looking at the word futile may have been that the author of the ReSPECT document may have felt that the act of DNACPR was futile rather than deeming the individual as such. According to Ardagh (2000) medical futility occurs when a suggested medical treatment is not expected to provide any substantial benefit for the patient. It is often discussed in cases where the treatment may not improve the patient's condition or quality of life.

One may suggest as a reader of the document that this could create the impression of ambiguity, which permits subjective interpretation as based on my personal experience. Therefore, this demonstrates the importance of highlighting the rationale for not implementing DNACPR on the document with a clear explanation of its intended meaning.

The terms 'learning disability' and 'Down syndrome' should never serve as a basis for making decisions on DNACPR, nor should they be used as the single or exclusive explanation for the underlying cause of death, as stated by NHS England (2023c). Moreover, although a learning disability is not usually life-threatening, individuals with such difficulties may be at higher risk of mortality due to comorbidities and other serious health issues (NHS England, 2023c).

The 2022 annual report of the Learning Disabilities Mortality Review (LeDeR) aims to investigate and learn from the preventable deaths among people with learning disabilities in England (King's College London, 2023). The report revealed that 74% of individuals who died in 2022 had a DNACPR in effect at the time of their death. Reviewers determined that this was accurately followed 63% of the time. This contrasts with a 61% occurrence rate in 2021.

Although ReSPECT documents are not legally binding, they should be included as a component of a comprehensive assessment in the best interest of the person (Wolff, 2017).

Supporting and encouraging involvement in decision making can promote empowerment for an individual, enabling person-centred and holistic approaches. Therefore, it is important to involve an individual in decisions that are in their best interests. The Mental Capacity Act (MCA) (2005) states that when an individual lacks the capacity to make a decision, any decision taken on their behalf must be done in their best interests. When determining a person's best interests, key principles include presuming capacity, supporting decision-making, allowing for unwise decisions, considering the individual's best interest, and choosing the least restrictive options for their rights and freedoms (MCA, 2005).

The Involve Me project developed by Mencap and the British Institute of Learning Disability (BILD) (2010/11) offers creative ways, such as guides and videos, to support prioritising people with profound and multiple learning disabilities to be involved at the heart of their decision making. Resources are available at: https://www.mencap.org.uk/learning-disability-explained/profound-and-multiple-learning-disabilities-pmld/pmld-involve-me.

Advanced care plans are important to adhere to if an individual loses the capacity to make certain decisions regarding their future care (Hamilton, 2017). Advanced care planning may include an advance decision that is a declaration of preferences regarding the medical and healthcare treatments an individual should wish to decline in the event they lose capacity in the future (NHS, 2022). This may include a decision not to be resuscitated under specific medical circumstances.

After consulting with my practice assessor, I was advised to approach the ward sister and request for the consultant to review and amend the ReSPECT document, providing a clear rationale for not implementing the DNACPR. The update was successfully authorised and completed on the same day.

In summary, reducing health inequalities is essential in the provision of support for individuals with learning disabilities, enabling them to overcome challenges and ensuring equal access to healthcare, thereby improving their chances for increased longevity and healthier lives.

Key considerations for nursing students to ensure that individuals with a learning disability receive fair and equal treatment include:

- Verifying if an individual has a hospital passport in place is vital as it provides essential information about their learning disability, healthcare and communication preferences. *It is recommended that individuals have multiple copies of these documents due to misplacement at hospitals.*

- Recognising early indicators of constipation can substantially minimise the risk of severe complications and avoid premature deaths in individuals with learning disabilities, who may have difficulty identifying these symptoms for themselves.

- The decision-making process for DNAR should take into account the advantages, disadvantages and challenges of CPR, together with the patient's wishes, values and beliefs. If you disagree with a DNACPR decision made by a doctor, you have the right to obtain a second opinion and a review.

Remember to: Always value judgements regarding the quality of life of individuals with profound and multiple learning disabilities.

Think box

Take some time to reflect, consider and think about the following:

1. **Departments not talking to each other – having to repeat information:**

   - Reflect on the impact of fragmented communication within health-care settings.

   - Consider the consequences of patients having to repeat their medical history and concerns across different departments.

   - Think about strategies to improve interdisciplinary communication and patient information sharing.

2. **Non-use of hospital passports by hospital staff:**

   - Reflect on the importance of hospital passports as a tool for providing personalised care to patients with learning disabilities.

   - Think about reasons behind the non-use of hospital passports by hospital staff.

3. **Advocacy services for patients with learning disabilities:**

   - Consider the role of advocacy services in empowering patients with learning disabilities to voice their needs and preferences.

   - Reflect on the barriers that patients with learning disabilities may face in accessing advocacy services.

   - Think about strategies to enhance the availability and effectiveness of advocacy services for this population.

   By Jose Ferin

References

Ardagh, M. (2000) Futility has no utility in resuscitation medicine. *Journal of Medical Ethics*, 26(5), 396–399.

Wolff, T. (2017) Time to ReSPECT personal resuscitation plans for adults? *BMJ* (356). Available at: https://doi.org/10.1136/bmj.j1634.

Hamilton, I.J (2017) Advance care planning in general practice: promoting patient autonomy and shared decision making. *British Journal of General Practice*, 67(656), 104–105. Available at: https://doi:10.3399/bjgp17X689461.

King's College London (2023) 2022 LeDeR report into avoidable deaths of people with learning disabilities. Available at: https://www.kcl.ac.uk/news/2022-leder-report-into-the-avoidable-deaths-of-people-with-learning-disabilities [Accessed 16 February 2024].

Mencap and Bild (2010/11) PMLD Involve Me. Available at: https://www.mencap.org.uk/learning-disability-explained/profound-and-multiple-learning-disabilities-pmld/pmld-involve-me. [Accessed 3 March 2024].

Mental Capacity Act (2005) Available at: https://www.legislation.gov.uk/ukpga/2005/9/section/4 [Accessed 18 February 2024].

NHS (2019) Learning Disability Mortality Review LeDeR programme. Available at: https://www.england.nhs.uk/wp-content/uploads/2019/05/action-from-learning.pdf [Accessed 11 November 2023].

NHS England (2022) Universal Principles for Advanced Care Planning. Available at: https://www.england.nhs.uk/wp-content/uploads/2022/03/universal-principles-for-advance-care-planning.pdf [Accessed 12 January 2024].

NHS England (2023a) Constipation resources for primary care teams. Available at: https://www.england.nhs.uk/publication/constipation-resources-for-primary-care-teams/ [Accessed 29 January 2024].

NHS England (2023b) Constipation campaign toolkit. Available at: https://www.england.nhs.uk/long-read/constipation-campaign-toolkit/ [Accessed 29 January 2024].

NHS England (2023c) Do not attempt cardiopulmonary resuscitation (DNACPR) and people with a learning disability and or autism. Available at: https://www.england.nhs.uk/long-read/dnacpr-and-people-with-a-learning-disability-and-or-autism/ [Accessed 18 February 2024].

NHS England (2023d) Learning from lives and deaths – People with a learning disability and autistic people (LeDeR) Action from learning report 2022/23. [pdf] Available at: https://leder.nhs.uk/images/resources/action-from-learning-report-22-23/2023/20231019_LeDeR_action_from_learning_report_FINAL.pdf [Accessed 19 February 2024].

Northway, R., Rees, S., Davies, M., Williams, S. (2017) Hospital passports, patient safety and person-centred care: A review of documents currently used for people with intellectual disabilities in the UK. *Journal of Clinical Nursing* 26(23–24), 5160–5168. Available at: https://doi.org/10.1111/jocn.14065

22

We are nursing in an imperfect world

Reflections on the importance of staffing and skill mix

Sonia Allibone

We are nursing in an imperfect world because learning disability nursing is shaped by inequalities, resource limitations and human fallibility. Learning disability nurses in inpatient services are middle management; they are responsible for the patients they care for and also responsible for the staff members that work alongside them. This makes the nurse's job difficult and they can find themselves in a position where they feel alone due to there being one nurse to 10–15 healthcare assistants. Nurses are responsible for making decisions and requesting staff to do different tasks. Nurses go from working alongside healthcare assistants one minute to working above healthcare assistants the next minute; this is where people struggle to differentiate positions. Although there are managers to manage wards and staff, they do not work 24/7 so the nurse is not always supported since ward managers are often attending meetings and dealing with operational duties. The further up a pay scale or the career ladder you go in healthcare the further you are from patient care so this is another weakness in inpatient services.

Inpatient services are often lacking in substantive staff; they rely heavily on temporary and agency staff, which causes inconsistency, ineffective communication and more work for the nurse to do as they are required to give new people inductions and guide new staff throughout their shift. Focusing on the physical and mental health needs of people with a learning disability is one part of our role; championing rights, independence, choice and inclusion for people with a learning disability is another, often overlooked but just as important, area. Unfamiliar staff impact on the care received by patients, as it is difficult for new staff members to fulfil patients' needs when they do not know the patients they are working with. This may also be difficult for staff members that are expected to work alongside

DOI: 10.4324/9781003341765-25

agency/pool staff members when they are in difficult situations and staff members are relying on each other for support; this often causes conflicts and yet again it falls on the nurse to resolve issues in this matter. When caring for people with learning disabilities and other complex needs, it is imperative to know the patients.

The nurse must always consider the skill mix of staff, which can be difficult when there is not a good mix of staff, therefore nurses need to know the staff's strengths and weaknesses. There is more expectation put on experienced staff to guide and lead agency staff. This puts pressure on staff and causes stress, and again can cause conflict amongst the staff team as working in a busy unpredictable ward staff need to feel safe and supported. When staff members are burnt out from work overload, they may receive no incentive or acknowledgement of their hard work, so they will go off sick or look for other employment. This is the cycle of workers in learning disability inpatient services that I have experienced.

Student nurses are sent to inpatient services; it is difficult for them to learn while there are staff shortages. This puts more of a workload on the nurse and the nurse can feel inadequate within their role as they do not have the capacity to fulfil all their duties. Students will struggle to get competencies signed off as they would feel uncomfortable to approach nurses that are stressed and busy. Each service where student nurses attend for placement should be given a list of duties to complete or have their own checklist/competencies that the student can complete while on placement. This gives the student some autonomy and will help them gain experience of the service. For example, it could be a task of: familiarise yourself with the immediate life support bag checklist located in the clinic room, look at the items used and identify them and their uses; check patients' drug cards and identify what medication is used, the uses, indications and doses, contra-indications, etc.

The most important job of the learning disability nurse is to promote their patients' well-being in all aspects of their life; this is called the holistic approach. This can feel overwhelming and difficult to achieve due to the supporting staff who are unfamiliar with patients' needs, not documenting information, not understanding people with learning disabilities, autism and mental health issues. The nurse relies on the care staff to pass information on, to ensure all food, fluid, bowel records are completed, to support and encourage good personal hygiene, eat and drink well, take part in activities, daily living skills and have good sleep hygiene, all of which promotes good health and wellbeing.

If staff do not have the correct training, knowledge and understanding they don't understand the importance of good record keeping and communication. The system of communicating can be very poor when there is an inconsistent staff team that always affects the patient's care. Yet learning disability nursing is a profession rooted in compassion, advocacy and evidence based practice. Learning disability nurses bridge gaps in care and adapt to these constraints.

It is important for the nurse to stand up for what is right and report staff's inadequate performance, or attitudes to their superior or management. Challenging these issues breaks the cycle of bad practice, inadequate care and does not allow for any negative cultures. The imperfect world does not diminish the value of learning disability nursing – it reinforces the necessity.

Quiz

1. **How does reliance on agency staff affect consistency and communication in caring for people with learning disabilities?**

   A) Improves consistency and communication

   B) Holds back consistency and communication

   C) Does not impact on consistency and communication

2. **What are the implications of inadequate staffing or inadequate skill mix of staff for patient care and continuity in an inpatient service?**

   A) Enhanced patient care and continuity

   B) No impact on patient care and continuity

   C) Compromised patient care and continuity

3. **How does a lack of familiarity among staff members impact on individuals with learning disabilities outcomes and person-centred care delivery?**

   A) Reduces patient outcomes and person-centred care

   B) No impact on patient outcomes and person-centred care

   C) Enhances patient outcomes and person-centred care

Correct answers:

1. C) Holds back consistency and communication

2. B) Compromises patient care and continuity

3. A) Reduces patient outcomes and person-centred care

By Jose Ferin

23

Medication and diet in individuals with a learning disability

Baldwin Ngambi and Lee Vessey

The use of medicines is the most widely used intervention in healthcare and can bring significant health benefits; however, medicines also have the potential to cause problems. Traditionally there has been a reliance on the biomedical model for patient care. Emphasis was solely on curing the illness and focusing on the biological aspects of the individual's needs (Ball, 2017), and therefore continued use of medication without considering the holistic factors affecting the individual. The needs of people with learning disabilities differ from person to person hence an individualised approach to care suits this group of people. In learning disability nursing the emphasis is on person-centred care, therefore getting to know the individual being supported through therapeutic engagement and a holistic approach. In recent years, the Moulster and Griffiths learning disability nursing model (2019) serves as a good practice framework to help learning disability nurses structure their work for more consistent care (continuity of care) and less conflict in the team, as well as improving understanding of the role of the nurse to other professionals and aiding decision making and goal setting (Pearson, Vaughan and FitzGerald, 2005). By using the Moulster and Griffiths model, learning disability nurses would be ensuring that nursing care is evidence based and person-centred (Ames, 2013), collaborative and reflective (learning from practice).

Improving medicine safety and optimising the learning from medication incidents reduces the risk of avoidable harm from medicines. And by reducing the number of unnecessary medications we can reduce this risk even further. So, with this in mind, we should be taking the lessons learnt by the STOMP initiative. Stopping the over-medication of people with learning disabilities and/or autism (STOMP) was established in 2016 to reduce the use of psychotropic drugs for challenging behaviour in people with a learning disability/autism and promote the development and uptake of alternative interventions such as non-pharmaceutical

DOI: 10.4324/9781003341765-26

(NHS England). Essentially it is about helping people to stay well and have a good quality of life. The NHS trusts have signed up to the STOMP pledge to proactively review psychotropic medications prescribed to people with a learning disability/autism. These psychotropic medications include antipsychotics, antidepressants, mood stabilisers, anxiolytics (benzodiazepines), sedatives and antiepileptics (MIND, 2024).

Psychotropic medications have a range of side effects that people with learning disabilities/autism will experience; however, due to communication difficulties in this population group it remains a challenge to reliably report unwanted side effects (Jenkins, 2000) despite appearing more sensitive to adverse side effects of psychotropic medications (Sheehan et al., 2017). These side effects include weight gain, high blood sugars, high blood pressure, high cholesterol, feeling tired and serious problems with physical health.

People with a learning disability who present with behaviours that challenge are more than likely to be prescribed psychotropic medication than those who do not have behavioural issues, in the absence of a formal mental health diagnosis (Niven et al., 2018). Moreover, researchers also found that prescribing can occur in the absence of other multidisciplinary team-based assessments that should serve to provide holistic support to meet the person's needs. There is a risk of diagnostic overshadowing which can potentially delay in diagnosis and access to appropriate treatment and care due to misdiagnosis and overprescribing. Nurses should be routinely conducting initial behaviour assessments/functional analysis of people exhibiting behaviours that challenge.

The learning disability mortality review programme (2020) (LeDeR) highlighted that one of the most frequently prescribed groups of medication were the anti-epileptic drugs (AED) group of psychotropic medications prescribed to almost half of all the people with a learning disability who had died prematurely. The nurse needs to be aware of such risk to people with learning disability.

The major cardiovascular disease risk factor globally is the burden of overweight and obesity and is even higher among patients with mental health disorders including patients with learning disabilities exhibiting behaviours that challenge, compared with the general population. Unhealthy lifestyles and unhealthy diets common among patients in inpatient settings, as well as the negative metabolic effects of psychotropic medications, could be major contributors to the burden. People with learning disabilities are likely to live in poor socio-demographic areas, be on benefits, not in employment, engage in unhealthy lifestyles and buy cheap unhealthy foods and fizzy drinks (high in sugars, saturated fats and processed), compounding the already existing risk that comes with overweight and obesity. The nurse should be actively involved in health promotion, advocating regular reviews of psychotropic medication, and using positive behavioural support plans to ensure optimal care to people with a learning disability.

A gentle nudge in the direction of a healthier lifestyle through education and awareness could prevent the need for many of the PRN medications being used by our patients today.

It is well documented that people with a learning disability suffer inequalities within healthcare throughout their lives, and this is exacerbated when the treatment they get could potentially be doing more harm than good (Emerson and Baines, 2010). Heart burn, acid reflux, bloating, indigestion, all are signs of a poor diet and nutrient deficiency in the body. Public Health England (2017) is just one source that tells us people with a learning disability tend to consume a very poor and sometimes limited diet, consisting of high sugar and processed foods. So it is of no surprise that they often exhibit nutrient deficiencies. Some of the side effects from nutrient deficiency are magnesium deficiency (cramping, headaches, stomach issues and constipation), Vitamin B12 deficiency (memory issues, brain fog tingling and numbness), Vitamin C deficiency (dry hair and nails, bruise easier, gives you fatigue and weakness) and zinc deficiency (hair loss, lack of alertness, loss of appetite).

The tendency is to prescribe medications, such as paracetamol, omeprazole or lansoprazole. These are proton pump inhibitors (PPIs). We should not be treating nutrient deficiency with PPIs that are full of sugar and carbs, which produces glucose, which causes an insulin spike. The main role of insulin is to regulate blood sugar levels and to store excess glucose in your body for energy. Excess glucose gets stored in the body as fat in the liver called glycogen. Between meals when your insulin levels are low, the liver releases that glycogen into the blood as glucose which gives us energy. But if we keep eating throughout the day, i.e. breakfast, lunch, snack, dinner and pudding like we do every day, we end up keeping our insulin levels high and we never give our liver a chance to burn off glycogen, so we stay in fat storage mode. Over time our cells will start to resist the insulin hence we become insulin resistant. All the symptoms we feel are the body's way of telling us we need to stop and pay attention.

The General Practitioner (GP) is the first point of contact for diagnoses, treatment and referrals. Other healthcare professionals who may become involved include: diabetic specialist nurses, endocrinologists, dietitians and pharmacist.

By educating the patients and staff around the effects of sugar and insulin on the body, it is hoped that they will be motivated to try to improve their dietary habits which could potentially decrease the number of medications they consume and improve their wellbeing. So the message is: consume less sugar and processed foods, and take care of your health.

Think box

Reflect on the following questions:

1. How do health inequalities manifest in people with learning disabilities, regarding diet-related issues? Think about the importance of prevention of ill health and health promotion, and the social determinants of health (Emerson and Baines, 2010).

2. Reflecting on best practice guidelines from NICE (2008) and the Nursing and Midwifery Council (2018), what strategies can learning disability nurses employ to address health inequalities and promote healthier lifestyles and prevent ill health for individuals with learning disabilities?

3. Consider the role of reasonable adjustments to accommodate the diverse needs of individuals with learning disabilities, especially concerning dietary choices and medication.

4. What are the potential negative consequences of a poor diet linked with overuse of medication for individuals with learning disabilities, and how can nurses advocate for holistic, person-centred care to mitigate these risks?

By Jose Ferin

References

Ames, S. (2013) Model followers. *Learning Disability Practice*, 16(8), 13.

Ball, E. (2017) Evolution of contemporary nursing. In C. Brooker and A. Waugh (eds) *Foundations of Nursing Practice: Fundamentals of Holistic Care*. London: Mosby.

Emerson, E. and Baines, S. (2010) Health inequalities and people with learning disabilities in the UK: 2010. Durham: Improving Health & Lives: Learning Disabilities Observatory. Available at: complexneeds.org.uk/modules/Module-4.1-Working-with-other-professionals/All/downloads/m13p020c/emerson_baines_health_inequalities.pdf

Jenkins, R. (2000) Use of psychotropic medication in people with a learning disability. *British Journal of Nursing*, 9(13), 844–850. https://www.doi.org/10.12968/bjon.2000.9.13.5512

LeDeR. Learning Disabilities Mortality Review: Annual Report 2020. Bristol University. https://leder.nhs.uk/images/annual_reports/LeDeR-bristolannual-report-2020.pdf.

Matson, J.L. and Neal, D. (2009) Psychotropic medication use for challenging behaviours in persons with intellectual disabilities: An overview. *Research in Developmental Disabilities*, 30(3), 572–586. https://doi.org/10.1016/j.ridd.2008.08.007

Mind (2024) The Big Mental Health Report 2024. https://www.mind.org.uk/media/vbbdclpi/the-big-mental-health-report-2024-mind.pdf

Moulster, G., Iorizzo, J., Ames, S. and Kemohan, J. (eds) (2019) *The Moulster and Griffiths Learning Disability Nursing Model: A Framework for Practice*. London: Jessica Kingsley.

National Institute for Health and Care Excellence (NICE) (2008) *BMJ* 2008; 336 doi: https://doi.org/10.1136/bmj.39505.641273.AD

Niven, A., Goodey, R., Webb, A. and Shankar, R. (2018) The use of psychotropic medication for people with intellectual disabilities and behaviours that challenge in the context of a community multidisciplinary team approach. *British Journal of Learning Disability*, 46, 4–9. https://www.doi.org/10.1111/bld.12206

Nursing and Midwifery Council (2018) Platform 2 Promoting health and preventing ill health. 2.1, 2.2, 2.3, 2.4, 2.5, 2.9.

Pearson, A., Vaughan, B. and FitzGerald, M. (2005) *Nursing Models for Practice*. London: Butterworth-Heinemann.

Public Health England (2017) National Diet and Nutrition Survey (NDNS) https://www.gov.uk/government/statistics/ndns-results-from-years-9-to-11-2016-to-2017-and-2018-to-2019/ndns-results-from-years-9-to-11-combined-statistical-summary

Sheehan, R. and Osborn, D. (2015) Mental illness, challenging behaviour, and psychotropic drug prescribing in people with intellectual disability: UK population based cohort study, *British Medical Journal*, *351*, h4326. https://doi.org/10.1136/bmj.h4326

Sheehan, R., Horsfall, L. and Strydom, A. et al. (2017) Movement side effects of antipsychotic drugs in adults with and without intellectual disability: UK population-based cohort study. *British Medical Journal Open*, *7*, e017406. https://doi.org/10.1136/bmjopen-2017-017406

24

Mental capacity, communication and advocacy for people living with learning disabilities

Olumide Dada

The National Health Service (NHS) Constitution states that all NHS organisations must offer comprehensive, high-quality services that do not discriminate between patients and are based on clinical needs. The Constitution states that all service users have the right to participate in healthcare planning decisions and management of their treatment (NHS Constitution, 2023). These emphasise that the NHS is constituted on the principle of patients' equal accessibility to healthcare. However, data has shown shortcomings in the NHS's efforts to achieve these objectives, particularly with people with learning disabilities (PWLD) (Maguire et al., 2022). The COVID-19 pandemic amplified the impact of health inequalities particularly regarding lack of access to care and care experience by people with a learning disability (PWLD). The Learning Disability Mortality Review (LeDeR) programme (2020) stated that around 71% of vulnerable adults with learning disabilities who had COVID-19 were placed on do not attempt cardiopulmonary resuscitation DNACPR (University of Bristol, 2020). These alarming figures attracted the attention of many reviewers who criticised this decision stating three major concerns: the process was inappropriate often lacking involvement from the individual, their family or those who knew them well; poor documentation; and people were placed on DNACPR because they had learning disabilities (CQC, 2021).

Similarly, my experience as a registered nursing degree apprentice while supporting a person living with a learning disability to his appointment at the general hospital suggests there is a need for learning disability nurses to amplify their voice in advocating and helping to reduce inequalities faced by this population group.

The name of the person is pseudonymised as 'Jack' to protect confidentiality following the Nursing and Midwifery Council (NMC) code (NMC, 2018a). While supporting Jack at his appointment at the general hospital, I observed the

DOI: 10.4324/9781003341765-27

qualified general nurse assessing Jack was directing questions to Jack's supporting staff rather than to Jack himself. I redirected the question to Jack using clear language, avoiding jargon and giving him time to respond at his own pace. Jack engaged well and was able to give direct consent and participated in his care. I also observed my action encouraged the qualified nurse to continue engaging directly with Jack.

My discussion with the general adult-trained nurse suggests that she was not familiar working with individuals with a learning disability and appeared to have an unconscious assumption that Jack may have lacked capacity to communicate effectively due to the diagnosis of learning disabilities. Shortage of staff and high workload would not even let her go through Jack's hospital passport. Research shows that there is a high shortage of nursing staff in the UK (Morgan, 2022), which has contributed to staff burnout (Al Ma'mari et al., 2020).

Collaborative working involves communication. However, individuals with a learning disability may express themselves in unconventional ways compared with the general population group who can articulate their needs (LACDP, 2014). Studies have argued that inadequate communication between patients and care professionals, and lack of awareness or training by staff or carers often contribute to delayed diagnosis and intervention for people living with learning disabilities (Segerlantz et al., 2020; Amara, 2023; Greaves et al., 2023). This indicates the impact of diagnostic overshadowing in contributing to the health inequalities experienced by individuals with a learning disability. The National Council on Disabilities (2022) argues that diagnostic overshadowing can negatively impact on the quality of care, leading to delays in diagnosis and treatment, unnecessary or unsafe care, and inequities in healthcare.

The Mental Capacity Act (MCA) (2005) states that professionals should assume a person has capacity unless every reasonable step has been taken without success and it is established that he or she lacks capacity. It is a legal requirement to make reasonable adjustments in removing any information and communication barriers so that individuals with a learning disability can participate in decision making regarding their health (Equality Act 2010). An act or decision made on behalf of such a person must be made in their best interest and be effectively achieved in a way that is least restrictive to their rights and freedom of action (MCA, 2005).

Similarly, the NMC (2018a) also emphasises the need for nurses to take reasonable steps to meet people's language and communication needs using an array of verbal and non-verbal communication methods. Disappointingly, recent figures from the NMC register show that between April and September 2023, there was a decrease of -0.2% in the membership registration of registered learning disabilities nurses with a total membership of 16,806 compared with an increase of $+2.4\%$ of registered adult nurses with a total of registered adult nurses at 601,805 (NMC, 2023). This data shows a decline in the number of new learning disability nurses, suggesting in turn a decline in the likelihood of individuals with a learning disability receiving specialist professional and person-centred support.

The current nursing education standards aim to bring a better understanding to all fields of nursing on how to support people with a learning disability (NMC, 2018b). But there is a need for the development of more inclusive packages of care that will ensure the care approach is always tailored to the specific needs and abilities of each person in this while we as future or qualified nurses continue to advocate for people with a learning disability.

References

Al Ma'mari, Q., Sharour, L.A. and Al Omari, O. (2020) Fatigue, burnout, work environment, workload and perceived patient safety culture among critical care nurses. *British Journal of Nursing*, 29(1): 28–34. doi:10.12968/bjon.2020.29.1.28. [Accessed 14 January 2023].

Amara, P. (2023) End of life care planning for people with learning disabilities: Nurses are key to ensuring that service users' wishes on end of life care are not rushed or missed. *Learning Disability Practice*, 26(6): 9–12. doi:10.7748/ldp.26.6.9.s3.

Care Quality Commission (CQC) (2021) report 'Protect, Connect, Respect – decisions about living and dying well'. CQC's review of 'do not attempt cardiopulmonary resuscitation' decisions during the COVID-19 pandemic. [Accessed 8 January 2024].

Equality Act (2010), Sec 20. Available at: https://www.legislation.gov.uk/ukpga/2010/15/section/20 [Accessed 9 January 2024].

Greaves, P.J., Grabrovaz, M., Browning, S., Gibson, A., Mandysova, P., Alderson. J. et al., (2023) Caregivers of people with learning disabilities and their experiences of communicating with healthcare professionals. *Learning Disability Practice*, 26(5): 25–33. doi:10.7748/ldp.2023.e2206. [Accessed 9 January, 2023].

Leadership Alliance for the Care of Dying People (LACDP) (2014) *One Chance to Get It Right: Improving People's Experience of Care in the Last Few Days and Hours of Life*. Available at: https://assets.publishing.service.gov.uk/media/5a7e301ced915d74e33f09ee/One_chance_to_get_it_right.pdf [Accessed 16 November 2023].

Maguire, D., Williams, E., Babalola, G. and Buck, D. (2022) What are health inequalities?, The King's Fund. Available at: https://www.kingsfund.org.uk/publications/what-are-health-inequalities#access. [Accessed: 1 March 2024].

Mental Capacity Act (2005) c.9. Available at: https://www.legislation.gov.uk/ukpga/2005/9/section/1 [Accessed 29 February 2024].

Morgan, B. (2022) NHS staffing shortages – The King's Fund. Available at: https://www.kingsfund.org.uk/sites/default/files/2022-11/NHS_staffing_shortages_final_web%20%282%29.pdf (Accessed 20 February 2023).

National Council on Disability (2022) Policy Framework. Health Equity Framework for People with Disabilities. Available at: https://ncd.gov/sites/default/files/NCD_Health_Equity_Framework.pdf [Accessed 29 December 2023].

National Health Service (2021) Giving someone power of attorney. Available at: https://www.nhs.uk/conditions/social-care-and-support-guide/making-decisions-for-someone-else/giving-someone-power-of-attorney/ [Accessed 30 January 2024].

The NHS Constitution for England (2023). [online]. Available from: https://www.gov.uk/government/publications/the-nhs-constitution-for-england/the-nhs-constitution-for-england [Accessed 20 February 2024].

The Nursing and Midwifery Council (2018a) The code: professional standards of practice and behaviour for nurses, midwives and nursing associates. Available at: https://www.nmc.org.uk/standards/code/ (Accessed: 18 February 2024).

The Nursing and Midwifery Council (2018b) Future nurse: Standards of proficiency for registered nurses. Available at: https://www.nmc.org.uk/globalassets/sitedocuments/education-standards/future-nurse-proficiencies.pdf [Accessed 1 March 2024].

The Nursing and Midwifery Council (2023), Registration Data Reports. Available at: https://www.nmc.org.uk/about-us/reports-and-accounts/registration-statistics/ (Accessed: 13 January 2024).

Segerlantz, M. Axmon, A. and Ahlström, G. (2020). End-of-life care among older cancer patients with intellectual disability in comparison with the general population: a national register study. *Journal of Intellectual Disability Research*, 64(5): 317–330). Wiley. https://doi.org/10.1111/jir.12721

UK Government (2014) Make, register or end a lasting power of attorney. Available from: https://www.gov.uk/power-of-attorney (Accessed 29 February 2024).

University of Bristol (2020) Learning Disability Mortality Review (LeDeR) Programme, Annual Report 2020. Available at: https://www.england.nhs.uk/wp-content/uploads/2021/06/LeDeR-bristol-annual-report-2020.pdf. [Accessed 5 January 2024].

25

A reflection on communication and the use of hospital passports within an acute hospital setting

Debbie Marsh

Whilst on placement in the West Midlands as a nursing degree apprentice I had the opportunity to support a patient to A&E (ED) via ambulance. Despite working in learning disability services for several years, attending A&E as a student was a new experience. What was immediately apparent was the lack of knowledge around people with a learning disability from the hospital staff, who spoke to myself and my colleague rather than attempting to communicate with the patient. This made me feel like the staff felt the patient wasn't there, as if they didn't matter. The danger of this is that the person isn't listened to themselves or that a holistic assessment doesn't take place, as hospital staff were reliant on information from us rather than the patient. I feel this approach is likely to make patients feel undervalued and not listened to. I offered nursing staff a copy of the patient's hospital passport. A hospital passport is a document that provides hospital staff with all the necessary information required to treat an individual with a learning disability in hospital (NHS UK, 2022). The hospital passport was taken from us and left at the nursing station (which we could see from the cubicle we were in), where it was not read by any of the staff and appeared to be dismissed as not useful. The doctor who came to see the patient again spoke to me as the nursing student and made no attempt to communicate with the patient. There were no attempts to use accessible information to support and promote effective communication with the patient. Accessible information is the use of any communication aid that is adapted to suit the needs of the individual as set out in the Accessible Information Standards, (2016). The doctor explained they were required to take blood from the patient. I advised that the patient would not allow this as they were hypersensitive to touch on hands and arms, but the doctor dismissed my requests for reasonable adjustments for the patient to have blood taken from another source on the body and made the attempt to cannulate. Reasonable adjustments are part of the Equality Act (2010), and are in

DOI: 10.4324/9781003341765-28

place to ensure that anyone with a disability has fair and equal access to health and social care services in the same way a person with no disability would access these services (NHS England, 2023). Accessing the hospital is often a barrier for people with a learning disability as they struggle to access services and appointments due to poor facilities and environments that are often too busy, crowded and so noisy that the person is not able to cope. Making reasonable adjustments could mean using a facility with better access, an environment that is less crowded or has better lighting, or accessing appointments at quieter times.

The patient refused the doctor's attempts to take blood. Fortunately, the head of A&E had heard the commotion and had come to investigate what was happening. I explained to this doctor the issue we were faced with, and they agreed this was not helpful for the patient and that we should explore other options and cannulate elsewhere on the body. The doctor went off and found an ultrasound machine; they explained they could find a vein in the patient's foot if we thought that would be a better and a more acceptable route for the patient. This doctor then spoke to the patient and explained what they were going to do and although the patient was non-verbal with profound and multiple learning disabilities (PMLD), the patient appeared to relax and, using low-arousal techniques and calming strategies, the doctor went ahead with the procedure, found a vein and inserted the cannula successfully. Low-arousal techniques and calming strategies include dimming lights in the areas of the room where they were not needed by the doctor; also, only the doctor talking to the patient one-to-one and taking the lead in this situation was beneficial in helping the patient to relax. However, having staff who knew the patient well was important to support effective communication and ensure the needs of the patient were met and at the forefront of all decisions made.

This low-arousal approach allowed the doctor to take blood from the patient successfully and find that the patient had an increased white blood cell count which can indicate an infection is present. Further blood samples were sent off to determine the type of bacteria causing the infection and then medication was administered via the cannula straight into the patient's blood as this is the fastest method to treat infections. According to the 2022–2023 LeDeR report one of the main reasons for premature and avoidable deaths in people with a learning disability is poor communication, delayed diagnosis, and a lack of understanding and awareness of people with a learning disability and their health needs. This is further backed by government guidance 'All our health' (2023), a resource for health professionals to prevent ill health and promote wellbeing as part of everyday care and support for people with a learning disability.

This experience could have been detrimental to the patient, exacerbating their fear of A&E and needles which would likely have a negative impact on the patient's health in the future and their trust of nursing staff could have been compromised. However, thankfully on this occasion the head of A&E was extremely helpful and understood the need to get things right for the patient. On reflection had this doctor not have been on duty the outcome for the patient would have been different – the infection would likely not have been found and the patient's health would have deteriorated. This doctor showed that effective communication, care and compassion was paramount in this situation and the treatment of the patient. This doctor demonstrated person-centred care, collaboration and adhered to the NHS's 6Cs of nursing (NHS England, 2012). It is really important to note that whilst this is a good example of how a person with a learning disability can have a positive experience in hospital, it should not be an exception or a one-off – this should be standard practice when accessing a hospital for all patients.

Lack of communication and trust in healthcare services are a common contributing factor to why people with a learning disability face health inequalities and inequities (Williams et al., 2022). Often all it takes is for medical staff to listen to the patient themselves, or people that know them well and know how to meet their needs, to change the patient's perspective and outlook on negative experiences and change them into positives. Doctors on the wards have a lot of knowledge – but although they are the experts they don't know everything, and nursing a person with a learning disability may be something they do not do very often. This is where learning disability nurses are vital to advocate on behalf of the people they support, to ensure they have a voice that is heard, to make sure reasonable adjustments are made so they can access the same healthcare services and receive the same treatment as anyone else who enters the hospital, without delay or judgement. Using hospital passports to document information that is important to the person will help staff care for them. These documents are invaluable: they give the person a voice, they aid communication and help to ensure people with a learning disability are supported in a way that meets their individual needs.

Think box

Reflect on the following questions for critical thinking about the nursing challenges related to health inequalities for people with learning disabilities and barriers they face in accessing and receiving healthcare services, exploring proactive solutions to address these challenges.

1. **Hospital passport not transferring between wards:**
   - Reflect on the implications of hospital passports not transferring between wards for individuals with learning disabilities. How might this impact on their continuity of care and patient safety?
   - Consider strategies to ensure the smooth transfer of hospital passports across different healthcare settings to support person-centred care and effective communication.

2. **Lack of use of reasonable adjustments, e.g. not having easy read information or accessible formats:**
   - Explore the barriers that contribute to the lack of use of reasonable adjustments for individuals with learning disabilities in healthcare settings. How does this impact on their access to information and involvement in decision-making processes?

- Discuss innovative approaches to providing accessible information and implementing reasonable adjustments to enhance the healthcare experience for individuals with learning disabilities.

3. **Lack of understanding and awareness about the needs of PMLD (profound and multiple learning disability):**

- Reflect on the challenges arising from the lack of understanding and awareness about the needs of individuals with PMLD in healthcare settings. How can healthcare professionals enhance their knowledge and sensitivity to effectively support this population?

- Discuss the importance of person-centred care approaches and multidisciplinary collaboration in addressing the complex needs of individuals with PMLD and ensuring equitable access to quality healthcare services.

4. **Not understanding that behaviour is often a method of communication:**

- Consider the implications of not recognising behaviour as a method of communication for individuals with PMLD learning disabilities. How might misinterpretation of behaviour impact on the assessment and management of their healthcare needs?

- Explore strategies for promoting a holistic understanding of behaviour as a means of communication and care for empathetic and responsive care practices among healthcare professionals.

By Jose Ferin

References

NHS England (2012), *Compassion in Practice: Nursing, Midwifery and Care Staff, Our Vision and Strategy*. Available at: https://www.england.nhs.uk/wp-content/uploads/2012/12/compassion-in-practice.pdf [Accessed on 7 March 2024]

NHS England (2016), *Accessible Information Standard: Making Health and Social Care Information Accessible*. Available at: https://www.england.nhs.uk/about/equality/equality-hub/patient-equalities-programme/equality-frameworks-and-information-standards/accessibleinfo/ [Accessed on 7 March 2024]

NHS England (2023a), *Learning Disability and Autism: Improving health; Reasonable Adjustments*. Available at: https://www.england.nhs.uk/learning-disabilities/improving-health/reasonable-adjustments/ [Accessed on 19 February 2024]

NHS England (2023b), Learning from lives and deaths: People with a learning disability and autistic people (LeDeR), *Action from Learning Report 2022/23*. Available at: https://20231019_LeDeR_action_from_learning_report_FINAL.pdf [Accessed on 7 March 2024]

NHS UK (2022), Support if you are going into hospital: Learning Disabilities, available at: https://www.nhs.uk/conditions/learning-disabilities/going-into-hospital/ [Accessed 19 February 2024]

Public Health England (2023), Learning Disability; applying All Our Health. Available at: https://www.gov.uk/government/publications/learning-disability-applying-all-our-health/learning-disabilities-applying-all-our-health [Accessed on 7 March 2024]

Williams, E., Buck, D., Babalola, G. and Maguire, D. (2022), What are health inequalities?, The King's Fund, original published in 2020. Available at: https://www.kingsfund.org.uk/insight-and-analysis/long-reads/what-are-health-inequalities [Accessed on 18 August 2023]

The last word for now…

Andrea Page, Samantha Salmon and Helen Jones

'In life it is the little things that can make the biggest difference.' In other words, the moments that often go unnoticed are the ones that truly matter to people with learning disabilities and those that care for them. In this book we have highlighted some of the negative moments that have led to a miserable life or even death; for example, the use of dismissive language and terminology used (being referred to as 'having attention-seeking behaviour', 'having challenging behaviour'); not responding to signs of health deterioration; through institutional discrimination towards individuals with a learning disability which occurs in pockets throughout the NHS, leading to a failure to attend healthcare settings, misdiagnosis, lack of appropriate care and diagnostic overshadowing. Mostly this book highlights those positive moments and the little things that often have gone unnoticed which are having a positive impact and which truly matter. For example, a reminder that we should all be saying or writing 'person with a learning disability' and that we should be ensuring that we use valuing language; the use of low-arousal techniques which can create a work culture of reflection and humility; and the useful resources, top tips and think points threaded throughout this book range from little things you can do to much bigger things. We have given you insight and, in our opinion, useful advice on, for example, how to help recognise pain, understand what is happening, how to provide structure and predictability, and introducing affective reasonable adjustments to help the individual in your care. Throughout this book almost every author has also stressed the importance of effective communication. They have provided you with ideas and resources which we hope you will remember and refer to time after time, so that your little things make the biggest difference and do get noticed because your care is recognised as being exemplary, or because you receive recognition from the individual, their family, their carers, your practice assessor, your personal tutor as making a positive difference.

What we have achieved in putting together this book is a focus and inclusion of people with a learning disability, through including their own voice, through family members speaking on their behalf, through case stories, through student/apprentice or professional reflection. This book covers key challenges faced by people with a learning disability and the way in which family carers, healthcare professionals and nurses across all fields of nursing can work together to improve

DOI: 10.4324/9781003341765-29

their quality of life. The book emphasises the importance of good health outcomes through:

- Better physical care for people with profound and multiple learning disabilities
- Awareness and understanding of key legal challenges and how nurses can support people to navigate correctly and smoothly through
- Awareness of conditions that are more prevalent or may present differently in people with learning disabilities and being aware of current and evidence-based practices within these.

Having this knowledge and these practical tips will give you the necessary skills to ensure that you are able to support and care for people with a learning disability and autistic people.

As editors we must thank all the contributors who have worked with us to make this book happen, especially when we were emailing asking people to commit to deadlines, fit writing in between full-time work, full-time study and family lives. We hope they are as proud of this book as we are.

It is important to remember the lives and the stories of Oliver McGowan, Tony Hickmott, Rachel Johnston, Thomas Rawnsley and Laura Booth. We ask that you tell others about this book and share the things that have stuck in your mind.

The main message from us is to really empathise with the people you are supporting and their loved ones. Imagine being in their shoes and how to promote person-centred practice in all areas – the nursing process or your own professional frameworks. As editors we want to leave you with a message from Paula McGowan as a mother and activist who has worked tirelessly to promote the Oliver McGowan mandatory training: 'All that it takes is empathy, vision and a little bit of time.'

Index

Note to index: page numbers in *italics* refer to information in figures; page numbers in **bold** refer to information in tables.